The Cure for Arthritis

*What Sufferers of Arthritis Need to Know
to Cure Themselves of the Disease*

S. H. SHEPHERD

The Cure for Arthritis

The Cure for Arthritis. Copyright © 2020. All rights reserved.

This book is for reference and informational purposes only and is in no way intended as medical counseling or medical advice. The author and publisher shall have neither liability nor responsibility to any person or entity with respect to any loss, damage, or injury caused or alleged to be caused directly or indirectly by the information contained in this book.

No part of this book may be used or reproduced in any manner whatsoever without written permission except in cases of brief quotations (less than three hundred words) embodied in critical articles and reviews.

The Cure for Arthritis

"The treasure which you think not worth taking trouble and pains to find, this one alone is the real treasure you are longing for." - B. Traven, The Treasure of Sierra Madre.

"The greatest danger for most of us is not that our aim is too high and we miss it, but that it is too low and we reach it." - Michelangelo

The Cure for Arthritis

To my mother, who suffered from arthritis most of her life, and was relieved of it only by her death.

Contents

Prologue	6
Preface	8
Introduction	10
Arthritis 101	12
Commonly Recommended Treatments	18
The Importance of Alternative Medicine	29
The Causes of Arthritis	66
How to Change the Situation	91
The Cure for Arthritis	121
Dangers to Avoid	129
Abiding by Nature's Laws	144
Salt	148
Distilled Water	153
The Blood	171
How to Be Your Own Doctor	176
My Story	193
The Cure and Longevity	214
Afterwards	219
Next Steps	220
In Closing	221
Bibliography	223
About the Author	228
Appendices	229
Index	237

Prologue

There is nothing glamorous or fashionable about having arthritis. To my knowledge, there has never been a main-screen motion picture featuring actors or actresses stricken with the disease.

Like sciatica and spinal stenosis, arthritis seems to be excluded from the list of human ailments that are commonly seen on the silver screen. A reason seems to be that more dramatic chronic diseases, such as heart disease, cancer of the organs and Alzheimer's disease, are widespread in our culture. Another is that it is easier to relate to people burdened by the more common woes of life, such as death in the family, divorce, financial disaster and traumatic injury, than it is to relate to people who have arthritis.

But anyone who lives with arthritis is intimately familiar with its pains, its limiting effects on the body's ability to perform simple, everyday chores and tasks, and the despair that it engenders, an unshakable feeling that the disease will never go away or get better.

Because there is no magic pill or silver bullet for arthritis, and no standard medical treatment that cures it, sufferers of arthritis face limited choices. They can pollute their bodies with pharmaceutical drugs to relieve the pains, undergo surgery for joint replacements or joint fusions, or they can learn to cope with their predicament. But none are desirable options.

I fought a losing battle with osteoarthritis in various parts of my body, including the hands, feet and spine, for over seven years. After spending a great deal of time and money on the various treatments commonly offered for arthritis, but which had little or no

The Cure for Arthritis

impact on my condition as far as I could tell, I learned that only when the underlying causes of arthritis are attacked that a cure possible.

Fortunately, there is a good deal of information now amassed about what actually causes arthritis. Unfortunately, much of it is not available through the popular media sources, including the Internet/Web, nor is it found in newspapers, magazines or on television. It is found in books about human health that explain how diseases and other health issues develop, and how they are cured through the greatest healing machine ever, the human body.

The information is also found in reports on objective clinical trials and studies that have been conducted on human health, some of which are published in the NIH Record, and in the personal experiences of many people who have suffered from arthritis but who have cured themselves of the disease by their own efforts.

It is from this wellspring of information and knowledge that the cure for arthritis is proudly presented.

Preface

I disagree with Linus, in *Peanuts*, who said, "No problem is so big or complicated that it cannot be run away from." You cannot run away from arthritis. You cannot eradicate it with medication, get rid of it through medical treatments that involve hospitalization and surgery, and you cannot overcome it with stimulants or depressants. You have to face it. You have to deal with it somehow.

The best way to deal with arthritis is not to resign yourself to a life of pain and disability, but to understand what causes the disease and take the proper steps that remedy the causes.

One of the causes has been right under our noses for as long as we have been living, and yet it has gone almost completely unnoticed.

Imagine a vine branch deciding to live apart from the vine. Could the branch ever grow leaf or fruit? Of course not. Yet, we are likewise interfering with the best use of the life we have by eating foods that are detrimental to our health.

Margaret Hills, who lived in Britain during the 1950s and 1960s, proved to everyone's satisfaction that arthritis is primarily caused by the consumption of acid-producing foods, such as the foods most commonly eaten in the Western world, and that when these foods are avoided and alkaline-producing foods eaten in their place, arthritic patients lose their pains and inflammation and recover from the disease.

The evidence against the foods that are most commonly eaten in this country and throughout the world is so overwhelming that it is surprising that anyone would continue to eat them, especially when there are so many other foods that have been proven to promote and sustain optimum health and reduce the chances of getting diseases and other health issues.

We need look no further for proof of the destructiveness of most of the diets of the world than the rising incidence of heart disease, cancer, kidney disease, diabetes and a host of other life-shortening sicknesses, some of which were unknown only a few decades ago. The same is true for joint-related diseases, such as arthritis, bursitis, ankylosing spondylitis, avascular necrosis and gout. All are on the increase in this country and in the world.

Introduction

No one gains health through wishful thinking. Proper steps must be taken to overcome arthritis or any other health issue. When the cause and effect relationship between the disease and what we are doing to ourselves becomes apparent to us, the best solution will then be known, as well as the proper steps that are needed to put it into effect.

Despite the many advances that have been made in modern medicine, commonly referred to as conventional or mainstream medicine, a cure for arthritis has not come forth. It is still considered by most doctors and most people to be an incurable, degenerative disease.

In what is becoming a perpetual logjam in disease cure and prevention, modern medicine does not have a cure for many other chronic diseases that afflict humankind, including heart disease, diabetes, kidney disease, the neurological diseases, such as Alzheimer's disease and Parkinson's disease, and cancer of the organs. But that does not mean that a cure for arthritis, or other diseases, does not exist. It only means that conventional medicine does not have cures for them.

Most of the treatments being offered for arthritis provide little or no long-term improvement for arthritic conditions because they aim at relieving the symptoms of the disease. not the underlying causes.

To cure arthritis, a new approach is required, one that recognizes the true nature of the disease, one that does not aim at palliation, but prevention and cure, one that instead of aiming at relieving the symptoms of arthritis, attacks its underlying causes. It is only when the underlying causes of arthritis are adequately dealt with that any real improvement in the symptoms can be expected.

This book describes how to cure arthritis and how to ensure the permanency of the cure. While intended for osteoarthritis, the cure is known to be effective against rheumatoid arthritis, gout and psoriatic arthritis, and may also be effective against other types of arthritis. It describes the many health dangers of our current ways of living and why they must be changed. It provides information of vital importance for the attainment of health and well-being in this century.

Eckhart Tolle tells us in his book, *The Power of Now*, that in every life situation there are three choices or options that are available to us. We can remove ourselves from the situation, we can change the situation, or we can accept the situation. This book provides the sufferer of arthritis with the practical know-how and knowledge required to change the situation.

Arthritis 101

Arthritis is a painful and debilitating disease that affects millions of people in the world today. Although not a killer in the sense of many other chronic diseases, including the top 10 leading causes of death in this country, arthritis causes persistent pain and inflammation, imposes limits on joint mobility (oftentimes severely), and directly affects a person's quality of life. It can lead to long-term disability, hospitalization and even early death. It is the nation's leading cause of disability.

Ask a doctor for a cure for arthritis and they will tell you that there is no cure. However, it would be quickly followed by advice on how the symptoms can be relieved through drugs, such as Nonsteroidal Anti-inflammatory Drugs (NSAIDs), corticosteroids and narcotics. In addition, orthopedic surgery, including joint replacement and joint fusion, are available.

Pain killers, especially those of the pill kind, appeal to our mindset because they're easy to take and require little or no lifestyle changes. However, medication for arthritis is intended to relieve only specific, localized symptoms. They do nothing for correcting the underlying causes of the disease. The same can be said for orthopedic surgery for arthritis. Even surgical removal of calcified deposits from the interstices of joints does not prevent the buildup of the deposits from occurring later on.

Osteoarthritis is the most common type of arthritis in the world. "Osteo" means "bone-related," and "arthritis" means "inflamed joints."

According to the Centers for Disease Control and Prevention (CDC), the nation's health protection agency, 30% of people aged

The Cure for Arthritis

45 to 64 years, and nearly 50% of people aged 65 years or older, have doctor-diagnosed arthritis. In number instead of percent, more than 50 million adults and 300,000 children in this country have arthritis (!). More than 8 million Britons have it, and who knows how many other people in the world are afflicted by the disease. Osteoarthritis, the most common type of arthritis, affects 27 million Americans. The CDC forecasts a rising trend for arthritis in this country throughout this century. The number of adults expected to have doctor-diagnosed arthritis in 2025 is 67 million.

Arthritis can affect any joint of the body, but commonly affects the most active weight-bearing joints, such as the hips, knees, hands, feet and spine. If left untreated, it typically gets worse, which leads to bone deformities and complete loss of joint movement, rendering its victims to a painful state of existence for the rest of their lives.

The Joints

The joints of the body are where two bones meet for the purpose of allowing them to move. The bones are not attached to each other, but the ends are normally covered with soft connective cartilage tissue and a lubricating fluid known as synovial fluid which the cartilage cells secrete. Cartilage acts as a cushion between the bones, and the synovial fluid provides a smooth, gliding surface for joint motion.

The Cartilage

Articular, or joint, cartilage functions to protect the bones from rubbing together and causing pain. It's a wear-resistant, smooth, nearly frictionless, load-bearing surface.

The Cure for Arthritis

Cartilage is composed of water, proteins and a type of protein fiber called collagen, which is the main component of cartilage (it is also the main component of ligaments, tendons, bones and skin). Collagen has great tensile strength. Collagen networks, or matrices, in joint cartilage provide the mechanical support and structural integrity needed to bear the stresses and loads imposed on the joints. Joint cartilage is known to be the site where osteoarthritis occurs.

Calcium and other mineral crystals are commonly found in synovial fluid samples of patients who are suffering from osteoarthritis. They are also found in the joint-articular cartilage, the articular capsule, and in ligaments, tendons and muscle endings. Fiber inflammation (fibrositis) may result from the deposition, as well as hardening of the tissues that surround the joint.

In a normal joint, there is a balance between the continuous process of cartilage matrix degradation and repair. However, when osteoarthritis exists, there's a disruption of the homeostasis or balancing process as catabolic processes cause more cartilage matrix degradation than the body can repair.

When the cartilage collagen matrix is degraded, loss of cartilage function occurs, which is what produces the pains and inflammation of arthritis.

If arthritis is left uncorrected, it worsens with time. As cartilage breakdown continues to occur, the body, in its self-healing process, tries to repair the loss and protect the bones from further ill effects. In its attempts at doing this, however, the bones at the edges of where the rubbing occurs may be built-up. This is what causes the bone deformities of arthritis, which are signs of advanced stages of the disease. The cartilage eventually wears away and the bones rub against each other causing severe pain and irreversible joint damage.

I have never found a listing of the root, or underlying, causes of articular cartilage collagen breakdown in the popular media. What I have found are varying opinions about what causes its deterioration, that is, what causes osteoarthritis. Many of the sources state that the breakdown is due to aging, or wear and tear of the joints, and/or accidents and joint injury, although other sources state that these are risk factors for OA, rather than causes.

Other risk factors for OA that are cited in medical studies about cartilage breakdown include obesity and genetics.

Many of the articles published on the Web regarding articular cartilage collagen deterioration indicate a need for continued medical research, which suggests that the cause, or pathogenesis, of cartilage breakdown is not well understood by the mainstream medical profession. Just three examples are two National Center for Biotechnology Information (NCBI) articles,[1] and a Nature Research Journal article.[2] It is also supported by the fact that mainstream medicine has not come forth with a cure for arthritis.

---

[1] By Carol Davila of the University of Medicine and Pharmacy, Gastroenterology Department, Emergency University Hospital, Bucharest, published in 2014, entitled, "Osteoarthritis Pathogenesis – a Complex Process that Involves the Entire Joint;" second article by Steven Bowman of the Department of Orthopedics, Augusta University, et al., published in 2018, entitled, "Recent Advances in Hyaluronic Acid Based Therapy for Osteoarthritis."

[2] By William H. Robinson, Division of Immunology and Rheumatology, Stanford University School of Medicine, et.al., published in 2016 in Nature, entitled, "Low-grade Inflammation as a Key Mediator of the Pathogenesis of Osteoarthritis."

However, as will be explained later in the book, many nutritionists and nutrition-minded medical doctors believe that foods and substances that are harmful to the body result in toxic acid and mineral deposition in the joints and tissues of the body, which cause articular cartilage breakdown.

Cartilage breakdown can also cause bone outgrowth or boney lumps to form in affected joints, which is known to cause a pointed outgrowth of bone known as a "bone spur" (osteophyte). When that occurs, the production of inflammatory agents increases, as does the swelling of the area around the affected joint.

Whenever something harms the cartilage or gets into the small spaces between the bones of a joint, or when something adversely affects the synovial fluid in the cartilage, the cushion effect of the cartilage is lessened or inhibited, which eventually causes the bones to rub against each other, resulting in the pain and inflammation of osteoarthritis.

Rheumatoid arthritis is caused by inflammation of the synovial fluid membrane, which results in excessive synovial fluid, leading to pain and stiffness. *Traumatic* arthritis is caused by a joint injury that damages the cartilage.

In years past, arthritis was known by doctors as rheumatism or gout. Rheumatism was the blanket term used to cover a wide variety of irregularities not limited to arthritis that involved pain and inflammation of the joints of the body. Today, we have, for example, the specific terms of osteoarthritis, rheumatoid arthritis, juvenile arthritis, psoriatic arthritis, gout, lupus and fibromyalgia.

"Nobody has rheumatism today, for the old "disease" has been run through a food chopper and so fragmentized that today we have a whole variety of "diseases" as substitutes for rheumatism. We have "neuralgia," "neuritis," "sciatica" (which is a neuritis), "fibrosis," "arthritis," "myositis" "bursitis," etc. Just as arthritis may develop in any movable joint and neuritis may develop along the course of any nerve, so fibrositis may develop in any fibrous tissue, myositis may develop in any muscular tissue and bursitis may develop in any bursa. "Itis" is a little Greek word meaning inflammation, which is used as a suffix. When added to the name of an organ or part, it indicates inflammation in that organ or part. Thus, all of these separate diseases in many different locations are but local inflammations. Their names do not seem to be important." - Dr. Herbert Shelton.

Ligaments and Tendons

Ligaments are fibrous connective tissue that attach bone to bone. Tendons are fibrous connective tissue that attach muscle to bone. The only type of arthritis known to affect ligaments and tendons is psoriatic arthritis, which causes swelling not only of joints, but of the surrounding tissue as well.

Statistics

According to a July 2007 Healthcare Cost and Utilization Project (HCUP) statistical brief posted on the Web entitled, "Hospital Stays Involving Musculoskeletal Procedures, 1997-2005," by Chaya Merrill, M.P.H. and Anne Elixhauser, PhD, the number of knee surgeries in the US rose by 69% between 1997 and 2005, from 328,800 to 555,800. Hip replacements rose 32% from 290,700 to 383,500. And spinal fusion surgeries increased by 73% from 202,100 to 349,400 per year. The majority of the procedures were likely performed to treat OA. In 2013, the national costs of arthritis were $304 billion overall. Of this amount, arthritis-attributable medical costs were $140 billion and arthritis-attributable lost wages were $164 billion.

Commonly Recommended Treatments

Many physicians, practicing therapists and chiropractors believe, in accordance with their medical training, that arthritis is a degenerative disease frequently affecting the hands and weight bearing joints of the body, and that it is primarily caused by wear and tear of the joints, accidents, injuries and joint misalignments.

Mainstream medicine places its emphasis on treating specific, localized symptoms of arthritis. The treatment strategies employed try to limit or slow down the progression of the disease.

Modern drugs are prescribed for relieving the pains and inflammation of arthritis. correcting one symptom or another, and surgical procedures are performed for relieving symptoms that cannot be controlled by medication or other treatments. Orthopedic surgery, such as a knee or hip replacement, and other procedures, such as arthrodesis (joint fusion), are typically offered for longer term and additional pain relief for patients unable to get the pain relief they need through drugs.

<u>Drugs</u>

Prescription drugs for arthritis include Nonsteroidal Anti-inflammatory Drugs (NSAIDs), such as the non-prescription pain relievers that include aspirin, ibuprofen (Advil, Motrin), Excedrin, Aleve, and also prescription kinds, such as diclofenac, celecoxib (Celebrex), phenylbutazone, and the Corticosteroids, which are hormones that include cortisone, prednisone, and methylprednisolone. Another class of prescription NSAIDs is cyclooxygenase (COX) inhibitors.

The Cure for Arthritis

Despite their ubiquitous use for treating the symptoms of arthritis, NSAIDs offer only short-term relief and come with risks and downsides.

A 2020 Web article entitled, "NSAIDs Cause Osteoarthritis," by Fred D. Arnold, NMD, states that numerous scientific studies have shown that patients who use NSAIDs to treat osteoarthritis have increased cartilage breakdown that leads to the need for joint replacements. It also states that it is the massive use of NSAIDs in patients with OA during the past forty years that has led to the rapid rise in the need for hip and knee replacements, as revealed in the HCUP statistical brief that was cited in the last chapter. In addition, it states that over 100,000 people are hospitalized for gastrointestinal (GI) bleeding and 16,500 die from NSAID toxicity each year.

As reported by the Annual European Congress of Rheumatology (EULAR) in 2018, NSAIDs that are used in the treatment of osteoarthritis enhance the risk for cardiovascular events, such as stroke, heart attack, and congestive heart failure.

NSAIDs may give pain relief that lasts a few months or even longer, but they are anti-inflammatory drugs that work by reducing the activity of the immune system, meaning that NSAIDs increase the likelihood of getting infections.

In a 2010 Journal of Prolotherapy article,[3] the author recommended that the following warning label be put on each NSAID bottle:

---

[3] by Ross A. Hauser, MD, entitled, "The Acceleration of Articular Cartilage Degeneration in Osteoarthritis by Nonsteroidal Anti-inflammatory Drugs."

"The use of this nonsteroidal anti-inflammatory medication has been shown in scientific studies to accelerate the articular cartilage breakdown in osteoarthritis. Use of this product poses a significant risk in accelerating osteoarthritis joint breakdown. Anyone using this product for the pain of osteoarthritis should be under a doctor's care and the use of this product should be with the very lowest dosage and for the shortest duration of time." - Ross A. Hauser, MD.

In 2015, the FDA published the following Safety Announcement concerning NSAIDs:

"The U.S. Food and Drug Administration (FDA) is strengthening an existing label warning that non-aspirin nonsteroidal anti-inflammatory drugs (NSAIDs) increase the chance of a heart attack or stroke. Based on our comprehensive review of new safety information, we are requiring updates to the drug labels of all prescription NSAIDs. As is the case with current prescription NSAID labels, the Drug Facts labels of over-the-counter (OTC) non-aspirin NSAIDs already contain information on heart attack and stroke risk. We will also request updates to the OTC non-aspirin NSAID Drug Facts labels. Patients taking NSAIDs should seek medical attention immediately if they experience symptoms such as chest pain, shortness of breath or trouble breathing, weakness in one part or side of their body, or slurred speech." – USDA, 2015.

Again, Dr. Hauser, in the above-cited article:

"One of the basic tenants of medicine is stated in the Hippocratic oath, "I will prescribe regimens for the good of my patients according to my ability and my judgment and never do harm to anyone." For doctors to uphold this statement in the treatment of their OA patients, it would necessitate the almost complete banning of the use of NSAIDs for this condition. If this does not occur, then most likely the exponential rise in degenerative arthritis and subsequent musculoskeletal surgeries, including knee and hip replacements, as well as spine surgeries, will continue for decades to come." - Ross A. Hauser, MD.

Despite these warnings, people continue to use NSAIDs to relieve arthritic pain. A GlobeNewswire *Fortune Business Insights* article, dated May 28, 2020, stated that the worldwide sale of NSAIDs was $15.58 billion in 2019, and is projected to reach $24.35 billion by 2027, although not all sales may be for OA.

Steroids, including corticosteroids, for arthritis are synthetic (man-made) drugs that can be taken orally or injected into a joint or bursa (the lubricating sac between certain tendons) or other soft tissue areas of the body. Like NSAIDs, steroids are anti-inflammatory drugs that work by reducing the activity of the immune system. Whenever the immune system is weakened, the likelihood of getting infections is increased.

Also, like NSAIDs, steroids may give pain relief that lasts a few months or longer, but they can cause many complications, including heart disease, kidney disease, tumors and cysts, acne, oily skin and hair loss, to mention only a few.

Another treatment commonly used for arthritis in recent years is hyaluronic acid, also known as hyaluronan (HA), a polysaccharide which is naturally found in the skin, and particularly in the synovial fluid of joints. As we age, the body's ability to synthesize HA declines, which, according to many medical professionals, is one of the reasons why more people get arthritis as they age. However, this view has been challenged since little is known about the biological mechanism(s) underlying the hyaluronan deficiency.[4]

The FDA has approved the use of HA in treating osteoarthritis. It can be administered orally, but is typically injected into the joint. Based on clinical trials of patients with knee arthritis, joint pain and inflammation improvement using HA is somewhat promising, but short-term[5].

Standard medical treatments for arthritis, whether they be drugs or surgery, have poor track records, especially in the long run. For example, a 2015 study on the long-term efficacy of NSAIDs in reducing OA pain[6] reported that, based on the results of clinical trials on over 4700 patients with knee OA, long term use of NSAIDs showed minimally important clinical change that did not reach statistical significance.

Pain killers appeal to our mindset since they're easy to take and require little or no lifestyle changes. Some of the medications on the market today for arthritis may even include what we believe are healthy ingredients. However, medication only addresses the symptoms of arthritis. Also, medication has risks and downsides for most everyone. The same goes for orthopedic surgery, as we will see.

The overall result of taking drugs for arthritis is that patients must

---

[4] 2015 NCBI article by Shuko Terazawa, Research Institute for Biological Functions Chubu University,Japan, et. al., entitled, "The Decreased Secretion of Hyaluronan by Older Human Fibroblasts under Physiological Conditions …"

[5] 2016 NCBI article by Mariko Oe, et. al, R&D Division, Kewpie Corporation, Japan, entitled, "Oral Hyaluronan Relieves Knee Pain: A Review."

[6] Kate L. Lapane, PhD, MS, et. al., "Effects of Prescription Non-steroidal Anti-inflammatory Agents on Symptoms and Disease Progression among Patients with Knee Osteoarthritis, published on a HCBI website.

cope with the toxicity of the substances that are prescribed for their condition as well as the condition itself. In addition, medications are often habit forming.

"The side effects of anti-inflammatory drugs cause at least 100,000 hospitalizations each year and some 10,000 deaths, according to official AMA figures. The actual figures are probably even higher as many adverse effects are often not reported. The chronic use of pain killers is now the leading cause of liver and kidney failure in the United States and perhaps in Europe." - Dr. Lawrence Wilson.

Surgery

The surgical options for arthritis include joint replacements for many joints of the body, including the hip, knee, shoulder and elbow. Joint fusion, a procedure for getting rid of the joint itself, is also available.

One of the most widely accepted surgical procedures for osteoarthritis is arthroscopic surgery, or arthroscopy. While typically used on the knee, it is also used on other joints, such as the shoulder, elbow, wrist, and ankle.

Arthroscopy allows doctors to see directly into the joint through an instrument called the arthroscope, a thin tube with a camera and light at one end. The arthroscope is used to find out how much damage is present in the joint. It can also be used to cut away debris, repair torn cartilage, or smooth out a joint where the surface has become rough.

The advantage of arthroscopy is that it does not require as much anesthesia or cutting as does other surgical procedures for arthritis, so the patient typically recovers quicker.

The Cure for Arthritis

However, according to a 2008 study published in The New England Journal of Medicine[7], researchers examined the effectiveness of arthroscopic surgery performed on the knee, and they came up with the following interesting results.

The research team, comprised of orthopedic surgeons, rheumatologists and physiotherapists, treated over an eight year period 178 patients having moderate to severe osteoarthritis of the knee, with an average age of 60 years. Eighty-six of the patients received arthroscopic surgery; the rest were treated with drugs, such as ibuprofen or acetaminophen. They were then tracked for two years to assess and compare the results. The result was that both groups of patients experienced similar improvements in joint pain, stiffness, and function, so that arthroscopic surgery was no more effective than drugs in treating arthritis of the knee.

The researchers concluded, "Based on the available evidence, we believe that the resources currently allocated towards arthroscopic surgery for osteoarthritis would be better directed elsewhere."

Another surgical procedure used for arthritis, including but not limited to osteoarthritis, is joint arthroplasty. This procedure replaces either the joint itself or parts thereof, such as the cartilage, by an endoprosthesis, or artificial device such as an

---

[7] The study, entitled, "Popular Surgery Provides No Relief for Osteoarthritis," which was conducted in London, Canada at The University of Western Ontario and Lawson Health Research Institute, showed that routinely practiced knee surgery using arthroscopy is ineffective at reducing joint pain or improving joint function for sufferers of osteoarthritis. The study was designed by the late Sandy Kirkley, an orthopedic surgeon specializing in arthroscopic surgery. It was coordinated by the Clinical Trials Group at Robarts Research Institute and conducted by orthopedic surgeons at the Fowler Kennedy Sport Medicine Clinic at London Health Sciences Centre.

artificial joint or another prosthesis. In other words, the procedure involves an implant. Joint arthroplasty is typically reserved for patients who have joint pain that cannot be controlled by other medical treatments such as drugs. Common examples of arthroplasty surgery for osteoarthritis, and for rheumatoid arthritis, is hip and knee arthroplasty, which is the surgical reconstruction or replacement of these joints. The terms joint arthroplasty and joint replacement are used interchangeably.

Osteotomy, or bone cutting, is also available. It is a surgical procedure for repairing damage to one or more areas of the affected joint. It does this by scraping away the bone, or areas of bone, that are causing the pains of arthritis. The procedure may be performed prior to, or in combination with, other types of surgery for arthritis, such as joint arthroplasty. Osteotomy sometimes adds a wedge of bone near the joint that is designed to shift weight off the damaged area (such as joint cartilage) to an undamaged area to reduce or relieve the pain of arthritis in the joint.

A type of osteotomy is arthrodesis, the surgical immobilization of a joint by fusion of the adjacent bones. Another term for it is joint fusion. This procedure is typically performed on smaller joints, such as those of the wrists and ankles, but is also performed on larger joints, such as the joints of the spine. Like joint arthroplasty, arthrodesis is typically reserved for patients who have joint pain that cannot be controlled by other standard medical treatments.

Sometimes, a small piece of bone, taken for example from the pelvis or tibia, is placed in the affected area to assist the fusion. Screws, wires or metal plates are used to close the gap within the joint. These parts stay in the joint even after it heals, and may result in complications that require additional surgery to correct.

The risks associated with surgery for arthritis include: bleeding in the joint, blood clots, nerve damage, infection, joint dysfunction, a later need for additional surgery, failure of the bones to fuse in the case of arthrodesis, failure of the bones to heal, bones that don't align as they heal, long recovery times, especially for joint fusion and arthroplasty surgery, and hardware that breaks in the case of arthrodesis surgery.

Other drawbacks of surgery for arthritis include the costs associated with the procedure and the hospital stay. Even for patients who are allowed to recover at home, the surgical procedures are performed in a hospital. Additional costs include post-op doctor visits, prescribed medication and the follow-up therapies that are prescribed.

As reported by many patients who have undergone surgical procedures for arthritis, the treatments have caused more suffering, disappointment, and inconvenience than the arthritis itself.[8]

Isn't it time that we ask ourselves whether we are likely to receive the best health care for our arthritis in healthcare centers and hospitals?

Perhaps the most significant drawback of surgery for arthritis is that it does not relieve the underlying causes of the disease, only

---

[8] For example, see the online 2020 Philadelphia Inquirer article entitled, "Medical Mystery: Why Was Her Arthritis Pain Worse After Surgery to Relieve It?"; the 2016 MDedge article entitled, "Less Symptomatic Patients Worse Off After Knee Surgery," the 2014 WebMD article entitled, "Common Knee Surgery May Boost Arthritis Risk," all of which deal with osteoarthritis, and scores of reports online regarding complications experienced after surgery for rheumatoid arthritis.

its symptoms, meaning, among other things, that recurrence of the pains and inflammation of arthritis after surgery is possible since the causes have not been dealt with. As revealed in many medical studies covering surgical procedures for arthritis on the popular media, even arthrodesis, or joint fusion, does not preclude the possibility of arthritis developing in nearby joints after surgery.

If the cause, or causes, of a disease – no matter what the disease may be -- are not addressed in treatments, then no lasting improvement in the symptoms of the disease can be expected.

Other Standard Medical Treatments

Other standard medical treatments for arthritis include narcotics, such as opioids, and radiation therapy. But these treatments also have undesirable side effects, and narcotics are known to be habit forming. In addition, these treatments address only the symptoms of the disease.

Summary

Despite the advances that have been made in the medical sciences over the years, modern medicine still considers arthritis to be an incurable, degenerative disease. Modern drugs are prescribed for correcting one symptom or another, but without effectively strengthening the overall state of health. Surgery may correct an arthritic condition for a time, but since it does not treat the underlying causes of the disease, it cannot be of any long-lasting aid for the condition.

The risks associated with surgery for arthritis are many, including joint dysfunction and the need for later surgery.

The Cure for Arthritis

As reported by many patients who have undergone surgical procedures for arthritis, the treatments have caused more suffering, disappointment, and inconvenience than the arthritis itself.

The treatments offered for arthritis are palliative, not curative, measures that provide little or no long-term benefit for arthritic conditions, although short-term benefit may be seen. It is only when the underlying causes are adequately dealt with in any treatment that any real improvement in the symptoms can be expected.

As stated previously, to cure arthritis, a new approach is required, one that recognizes the true nature of the disease, one that is not aimed at palliation, but prevention and cure, one that does not treat its symptoms but attacks its underlying causes.

Arthritis is curable. It is only what cannot be cured that must be endured.

The Importance of Alternative Medicine

Before beginning the discussion about alternative medicine treatments for arthritis, some observations about the standard medical treatments described in the last chapter are warranted.

Standard medical treatments for arthritis, as well as for most other diseases and health disorders, rely heavily on achieving health through drugs. For arthritis, take pain killers. For headaches, take aspirin or a similar product; for stomachaches, take antacids; for infections, take antibiotics; for constipation, take laxatives; for cancer, take chemotherapy or radiation therapy. But even considering drugs like penicillin which can halt the spread of a disease, drugs do not possess the ability to cure[9], and risks are associated with taking all drugs. Also, drugs have been known to lodge in the system for decades after their use[10].

Permanent cures of diseases by mainstream medicine are rare[11]. It is believed that many of the cures that are attributed to mainstream medical treatments would have occurred naturally without them.

---

[9] Healing does not come from drugs. It comes from natural bodily processes as will be shown in this book, such as self-cleansing or detoxification that remove accumulated toxins, obstructions and acidosis from the body, from rest, and from providing the body with the nourishment it needs.

[10] From the book, Prof. Arnold Ehret's Mucusless Diet Healing System: Annotated, Revised, and Edited by Prof. Spira.

[11] For example, the average cure rate for all types of cancer by mainstream medicine, except for skin cancer, is 17% per G. Edmond Griffin's book, World Without Cancer. It is believed to be more like 6% per Rich Anderson's book, Cleanse & Purify Thyself. A 2019 American Cancer Society Web article states that most cancers cannot be cured, but some can be controlled for months or even years. A cancer.net article sponsored by the American Society of Clinical Oncology (ASCO) states that chronic cancer is cancer that cannot be cured.

The Cure for Arthritis

Modern drugs are prescribed for arthritis for correcting one symptom or another without effectively strengthening the overall state of health. However, the body is an integral organism consisting of many parts, with every part connected with every other part. All parts of the body receive the same blood and lymphatic fluid supply to support its needs. No one part can be diseased and the rest be healthy. As such, all talk of arthritis being localized is nonsense, and implies an ignorance of what constitutes the true nature of the disease.

Thousands of hospitals worldwide conduct surgical procedures around the clock for orthopedic joint replacements and removal of bone spurs. Yet, as shown in the last chapter, the procedures do not address the root causes of the conditions. Also, surgery can result in further complications, such as infections, joint dysfunction and the need for more surgery. Surgery is also a very expensive option.

Many nutritionists have known for years that unless dietary change is instituted as part of the post-op treatment program, the same conditions that surgery was intended to remedy may reoccur after surgery.

As mentioned previously, a new approach to curing arthritis is required. The approach that is needed is a wholistic approach. Alternative medicine, sometimes called complementary or naturopathic medicine, is a proven system of healthcare that views the body as the integral, whole organism that it is.

Alternative medicine uses natural methods for healing diseases. Many cases of advanced arthritis, including rheumatoid arthritis as well as osteoarthritis, have been completely cured through alternative medicine treatments.

The Cure for Arthritis

The medically trained and licensed practitioners of alternative medicine may be found in naturopathic clinics or institutes, the most renown of which are in Sweden, Germany and the US. They routinely heal patients who come to them for treatment. However, many people have found that alternative medicine treatments work very effectively at home, and that much time and money can be saved by not visiting a naturopathic clinic, or making an appointment with a local alternative medicine practitioner.

According to Naturopathic Medicine Doctors (NMD) and nutritional experts, including those whose books are listed in the Bibliography, local treatments are harmful to the entire body, not only the part or parts that may be displaying the symptoms. They contend that almost all attempts made by mainstream medicine to cure diseases are not successful in a true sense, but can, at best, only forestall the diseases from taking over and killing the patients in the short term.

A principle of naturopathic healing is to provide the body with the nutrients and other essentials it needs to enhance the body's self-cleansing process, and deprive the body of foods and substances, including drugs, that thwart the process. The body's self-cleansing process is always at work, but when the body is properly cared for in the ways that abide by the laws of Nature, the process ramps into high gear and can heal whatever is wrong with the body.

The diseases that have been cured by naturopathic medicine run the gamut, from heart disease to cancer of the organs, to multiple sclerosis to paralysis, and, as mentioned above, advanced cases of arthritis. Many of the cures have been without precedent. Many clinical trials and dietary studies have been conducted on the efficacy of these cures, and some are cited later in this chapter.

The Body

The body is a marvelously powerful healing organism capable of healing itself of diseases, restoring to health any ill-health condition and releasing its rejuvenating powers into action, but only if it is properly cared for.

When supplied with the life-supporting nourishment and other pro-health things that it needs, the body can remain in optimum health for much longer than the average human lifespan. It is designed for stupendous feats and deeds, as we observe throughout the world. The body's amazing resilience and its many capabilities far out-marvel anything made by humankind. Yet, in many ways it is fragile and utterly dependent on its caretaker for its needs.

The healing powers of the body are fully at work when we live in concert with the laws of Nature. But when we depart from Nature's laws by putting foods in us that harm the body, or do other things that are bad for health such as depriving the body of adequate exercise, sunshine, fresh air and rest. we court disaster in the form of disease or some other troublesome health issue. However, if we understand the laws of Nature and abide by them, illness and disease are vanquished by the body's inherent life-promoting and life-sustaining powers.

Anyone who has a health disorder, such as arthritis, has it for a reason. When the cause and effect relationship between a health issue and what we are doing to ourselves becomes apparent to us, the best solution will then be known, as well as the proper steps that are needed to put it into effect

One's overall state of health can often be determined from the answers to a few simple questions. For example, how many bowel movements per day are had? What types of foods have been, and are being, consumed, and for how long? What types of supplements are being taken and for how long? Is medication taken, and if so, what types and for how long? The answers to questions such as these provide important clues as to what is causing the health disorder or disease, and also what steps would likely remedy or cure it.

Some of the alternative medicine treatments employed for arthritis are described below. Instead of using drugs or medical intervention, such as hospitalization and surgery, naturopathic cures work with nature in ways that address the underlying causes of the disease and allow the body to heal itself. The treatments include depriving the body of what is causing it harm, and giving the body what it needs to heal itself, which are completely different from the commonly recommended treatments for arthritis, and are the very opposites of what many of us are doing to ourselves.

From a nutritionist's and an alternative medicine practitioner's viewpoint, many diseases that afflict us, including arthritis, are the result of either an unwitting ignorance of the unalterable laws of Nature, or a willful refusal to abide by these laws.

"Man's health or his disease of every description, directly result from food intake. His state of mind may be a contributing factor, but the fall of mankind in the final analysis is "sin of diet." The real physiological cause of all evils, especially the physical ailments of mankind can be traced directly to the present day accepted diet of civilization." - Arnold Ehret, *Rational Fasting and Roads to Health and Happiness.*

Avoiding Foods and Substances That Are Harmful to the Body

Many of the foods commonly eaten in this country are harmful to the body because they are linked to sickness and disease.

The Cure for Arthritis

People in this country should be the healthiest people on earth. It certainly seems that way since there are now more varieties of health-promoting foods available than ever before, and many of them organically grown. But we are not the healthiest people because of our preferences for artificial, man-made foods and drinks, our giving way to cultural norms and traditions about foods, and our unwillingness, even refusal, to abide by Nature's laws that govern health and well-being.

Many people believe that they are living healthy lives, but their diets are wholly lacking in nutrients and enzymes. Poor nutrition contributes to an acidic blood condition. Over time, this condition causes a buildup of hard acid deposits in the joints and tissues of the body, which is one of the causes of the chronic symptoms of arthritis, as we will see.

There is more scientific information available to us right now about how foods and nutrition affect health and well-being than ever before. Almost everyone is, at least peripherally, aware of some of this information. The information strongly suggests that cures for diseases, and lesser ailments of which the human race is susceptible, are available. Many dietary studies and clinical trials conducted on human health closely link health disorders to faulty dietary practices, practices that cause internal poisoning when the tissues of the body become congested with acidic and toxic wastes due to the foods that are commonly consumed.

Every day we witness the affects that these foods have on us. It is no secret that sickness and disease continue to plague us despite the billions of dollars of federal, state and private funds that are spent each year trying to find cures for our diseases, including heart disease, cancer and the other life-shortening and disabling diseases.

The Cure for Arthritis

It seems like everyone knows someone who is suffering from a health issue. Most of us have come to accept sickness and disease as a normal part of life. But nutritionists have been telling us for years that these things do not happen by chance, but are caused by the foods we eat.

Many of us continue to eat just as we did last year and the year before because of our habits. Another reason is that we have been culturally indoctrinated to believe that certain foods, such as meat and dairy products, sugary foods and drinks, and refined and processed foods, are good for us. Both pressures are reducing our numbers rapidly. Eating foods that we grew up on is not working.

People who eat the traditional American diet are nutrient deficient. This deficiency has been shown to be the cause of a number of serious health problems. To make up for the mineral-starved and vitamin-starved foods now being produced, many people take multivitamin/mineral supplements on the advice of their doctors. Billions of dollars are spent each year in America alone on these supplements.

Unfortunately, most of the multivitamin/mineral supplements are inorganic substances that cannot be utilized by the body. Studies have shown that these supplements provide little, if any, benefit to human health. See Web articles, such as from searching on "multivitamin/mineral supplements." It is also discussed in books by Dr. Ann Wigmore (see Bibliography), among others.

The cells of the body can only utilize minerals that are in organic form, which is one of the reasons why plant foods are so important to us. Plants convert inorganic minerals found in the soil and water into organic form that is readily assimilated by the cells of the body.

The Cure for Arthritis

"Inorganic minerals are rejected by the cells of the body, which, if not evacuated, can cause arterial obstructions and even more serious damage." - Norman W. Walker, *Water Can Undermine Your Health.*

Many nutritionists, including Dr. Ann Wigmore and others whose books are listed in the Bibliography, believed that arthritis was caused by eating foods that are harmful to the body, foods that cause toxic hard acids to be deposited in the tissues and joints of the body.

"Most problems with arthritis in its many forms, insofar as our experience indicates to date, are definitely related to diet – the foods, drinks and chemicals that enter the body through the mouth." - Dr. Norman F. Childers, *Arthritis - Childers' Diet That Stops It!*

Excitotoxins are substances added to processed foods and beverages for the purpose of stimulating brain neurons. For years, the food industry has designed food products to titillate the taste buds and activate the reward centers of the brain. The diverse chemicals that are used for these purposes include excitotoxins. The term was popularized by Dr. Russel Blaylock in his book, *Excitotoxins, The Taste that Kills.* As stated in the book, these substances are found in almost all processed foods. Excitotoxins include monosodium glutamate (MSG)[12], aspartame (used in artificial sweeteners), cysteine (used in breads), hydrolyzed protein, and aspartic acid. These substances can stimulate brain neurons so severely that they are killed, resulting in varying degrees of brain damage.

---

[12] According to Blaylock's book, the food industry is on a quest to disguise MSG in foods. A list of common additives that contain MSG is found in the book.

The Cure for Arthritis

Remember that piercing headache you got the last time you ate Chinese food? It was probably due to the MSG used on the food. The Web adequately covers the dangers of MSG, for example, do a search on "msg in foods."

As of this writing, there are no regulations requiring the food industry to test its products for whether they cause brain damage or food addictions.

The deliberate tampering of foods to increase taste appeal at the expense of harming the body, while attesting to the inventiveness and ingenuity of the American spirit, typifies how low we have sunk in manipulating foods for financial gain. I recommend Dr. Blaylock's book to anyone. It includes a list of chemicals that should be tacked to our kitchen walls. It will make you check the foods labels all over again.

It is entirely possible that the causative factor, or at least a major contributing factor, to the sharp rise in brain diseases in our culture, including dementia and other neurological disorders found in people, is the continued use year after year of food products that contain excitotoxins.

Dr. Ann Wigmore in her book, *Be Your Own Doctor*, states that inorganic salts get deposited in the joints of the body and cause arthritis. She healed herself of arthritis by eliminating table salt from her diet and going on a whole plant food diet.

Even members of the mainstream medical profession have implicated table salt with the high incidence of high blood pressure and kidney problems in the Western world. Table salt is unnatural, highly-refined salt. It has been heat treated to very high temperatures which alters the chemical structure of the salt. The salt is then bleached white and combined with anti-caking agents, fluoride, dextrose, aluminum hydroxide (to improve its pour-ability) and preservatives. Aluminum is widely recognized as a neurotoxin and a potential cause of Alzheimer's disease. An easy way to recognize refined salt is its bleached white color.

Other salts are commonly available today that have not been refined and subjected to high temperature heat treatment. These are the natural sea salts which are salts that come from evaporating sea water by the heat of the sun. Their chemical structure has not been altered. Natural sea salt does not contain man-made additives or ingredients, but is pure, unadulterated salt.

On a whole plant food diet. there is no lack of mineral salts for electrolyte health. If additional salt is desired because of worries about not getting enough salt, then natural sea salt should be used. Beware, however, that if "Sea Salt" is listed as an ingredient in a food product, then it is most likely refined sea salt, not natural sea salt. This is explained in the chapter on "Salt." If it is natural sea salt, the brand name of the sea salt, such as Celtic Sea Salt or Himalayan Sea Salt, will be listed.

Typically, the packaged shaker "sea salt" found in most supermarket aisles is bleached white in color, which reveals that it is refined salt. Natural sea salt is not bleached white but has a greyish or pinkish cast to it.

Organic minerals, the minerals we get from eating plant foods. are not deposited in the tissues and joints of the body, but are fully utilized by the cells of the body for their regeneration.

"The bottom line is this – no matter where or how on earth it comes from, if salt is not first transformed by plants from inorganic sodium into organic sodium, it can't be properly absorbed by the body." - Paul C. Bragg, *Water, The Shocking Truth That Can Save Your Life.*

For more information about salt, see the chapter on "Salt."

<u>Foods that Promote and Sustain Health</u>

Proper diet is the single most important alternative medicine cure for arthritis. Improvements in any arthritic condition can be said to begin when a common, or ordinary, diet is replaced by a healthy diet consisting of whole plant foods.

"In food lies 99.99% of the causes of all disease and imperfect health of any kind. Consequently, all healing, all therapeutics will continue to fail as long as they refuse to place the most important stress on diet." - Arnold Ehret, *Mucusless Diet Healing System.*

To be healthy today requires more than just limiting the amount of saturated fats in the diet or having a salad several times a week and getting proper exercise. It requires knowledge of foods and nutrition, a knowledge that many people simply do not have. We need to educate ourselves about foods and nutrition, and apply the storehouse of information that has been gained by nutritionists and nutrition-minded medical doctors over the years to solve more of our health problems.

By choosing to ignore the vast amount of information that has been gained in the health field which proves that diseases and a host of lesser human ailments are caused by commonly eaten foods, many of us are sacrificing our health for eating habits and food cravings. But the remarkable truth is that eating habits can be changed even when food cravings exist, and that everyone is capable of changing their diet in enlightened self-interest.

The Cure for Arthritis

The best diet is one that meets the energy and nutrient needs of the body and produces the least negative effects, such as toxicity, acidity, and constipation. For most people, it means a diet consisting of a large volume of fresh, whole fruits and vegetables to meet the body's nutrient needs, and enough concentrated foods, such as nuts and seeds, to meet the body's energy needs.

Whole plant foods are different in many ways from other foods. Apples, when planted in the soil, produce additional apple trees. Raw nuts planted in the ground produce other nut trees. Even a harvested potato when planted yields at least another potato plant. But many of the foods that are commonly consumed have been devitalized by heat treatment. Cooking destroys the life force properties that are in foods. Plant a cooked bean or tomato, or a roasted nut, in the ground and it will not sprout. Cooked foods, including refined and processed foods, do not promote or sustain health, but are harmful to the body.

Contrary to the tenets of mainstream medicine, nutritionists believe that disease is a rational process of the body attempting to cure itself of excess acid or toxic waste that it should not have accumulated. The main cause of this accumulation is faulty diet which creates acidity or toxicity in the body and causes constipation which, in turn, causes unfriendly bacteria to proliferate inordinately in the waste material that results in blood poisoning by the toxins that are thereby produced. In either case, the primary cause is improper diet.[13]

Bear in mind, however, that no cure can be expected to work while eating habits are constantly counteracting the cure.

---

[13] For more information, see the book, *The Powers that Heal*, which is listed in the Bibliography.

The Cure for Arthritis

Not everyone has the same nutritional requirements. But the body requires similar things for health and wellness, and we are all very much alike in numerous ways, having the same basic needs, the same general physiology, the same susceptibility to biological disharmony, the same susceptibility to many illnesses, and we share many of the same stresses, worries and fears that can influence our state of health. Nutritionists, whose voices have not been heard as much as those of ordinary diet proponents, have been telling us for years that ill-health and diseases of all types spring most often from one common source, namely, poor dietary practices.

The body requires a variety of nutrients, and enzymes to break down the nutrients, but ordinary diets, such as the Standard American Diet, cannot provide these things. According to nutritionists, including those who books are listed in the Bibliography, a whole food diet, such as the raw vegan diet (described later in the chapter on "How to Change the Situation"), provides the body with the nutrients and enzymes it needs to prevent toxic acid buildup, and rids the body of its toxins better than any other food regimen.

"Most persons are tired because their body lacks enzymes. The food they eat cannot be utilized constructively but is turned instead into toxins, poisons which lead to sickness. Enzymes, apparently, are the key to longevity; they seem to neutralize the basic causes of aging and enable the body to retain its youthful qualities." - Dr. Ann Wigmore, *Be Your Own Doctor.*

While many fad diets claim to be the best yet for health, there is one way of eating that guarantees long-lasting health benefits, and that is the whole plant food diet. It is a complete shift in eating habits away from lifeless, cooked foods to living plant foods, the only foods that have life force properties that both God and Nature intended for us to receive, which support all bodily functions and have the nutrients and enzymes the body needs to heal itself and sustain itself in health.

Additional Observations About Health and Diet

Nutritional experts and nutrition-minded doctors stress that sickness and disease cannot exist in a body that has cleansed itself of acidic and toxic wastes by the powers of living, whole plant foods, the foods that are most conducive to human health, the foods that have the powers to heal.

It has been my experience and observation that we are more than capable of causing our own sicknesses. We unwittingly bring sickness and disease upon ourselves through dietary practices that are contrary to the laws of Nature. As stated above, the body requires a variety of nutrients to keep itself in health, but seldom finds them in the foods that are commonly eaten. It requires enzymes for proper digestion, but they are destroyed by heat, and almost all refined and processed foods are heat treated. The natural law of cause and effect determines the outcome, which is ill-health.

The dangers of eating cooked foods is discussed in more detail in the chapter on "Dangers to Avoid."

A whole plant food diet enables us to heal ourselves of diseases and prevent them from taking root in the body, all due to the cleansing and rejuvenating actions that raw plant foods have on us.

To avoid the hazards that have been described, and more (I'm sure I haven't mentioned all of them) we should eat the foods of a whole plant food diet, which are raw (uncooked) plant foods. This

The Cure for Arthritis

is what nutritional experts have been telling us for years, as documented in their books listed in the Bibliography.

Today's real need is not another low-carb, high-protein diet, or an end to global warming (which appears to be mainly caused by the extensive deforestation to clear space for cattle and feed crops). Today's real need is self-education about foods and nutrition.

Typically, people resort to doctors when they don't know what else to do. But by simply utilizing the Web/Internet, as well as the information that is contained in books that are available to most people, many health concerns can be thoroughly investigated, and the proper treatments determined, without seeing a physician.

"But the foods which you eat from the abundant table of God give you strength and youth to your body, and you will never see disease. For the table of God fed Methuselah of old, and I tell you truly, if you live as he lived, then will the God of the living give you also long life upon the earth as was his." - Attributed to Jesus, *The Essene Gospel of Peace, Book One.*

Cider Vinegar

The importance of cider vinegar, or more precisely, apple cider vinegar (ACV), in relieving arthritic conditions has been recognized for years in the US and Europe. The use of ACV in treating arthritis is based on its ability to dissolve back into the bloodstream for their elimination the calcium deposits that have formed in the joints and tissues of the body.

Dr. D.C. Jarvis, a Vermont physician, was a famed proponent of ACV to cure arthritis. He explains in his two books, *Folk Medicine*, and *Arthritis & Folk Medicine*, how arthritis develops from a buildup of calcium in the joints and tissues of the body from foods and drinks that are ingested. Dr. Jarvis successfully treated many arthritic patients with the treatment and prevented himself from getting arthritis by it. He lived to be 85.

Dr. Jarvis recommended taking 1-2 tablespoons of ACV and 1-2 tablespoons of honey in a glass of water twice daily, at or between meals, to rid the body of its unwanted calcium deposits. The honey makes the drink more palatable, but honey has health benefits of its own, including being rich in organic minerals, such as potassium. Nutritionists tell us that potassium helps to metabolize calcium.

Dr. Jarvis observed the various ways that Vermonters used ACV to remove calcium deposits from their maple syrup sugar-house kettles.[14] The water added to the kettles is very rich in calcium due to the high calcium content of the Vermont soil. When the mixture is boiled, it leaves hard calcium deposits on the inside of the kettles which thickens in time, thereby reducing the effectiveness of the kettle to boil the mixture. To correct the problem, they add ACV to the kettles to remove the deposits. The proportion used is one cup of ACV per quart of water. The acid in the cider chemically attacks the calcium deposits, dissolving them and returning them back into solution. The result is clean kettles. The same treatment is used to dissolve calcified scale from furnace water tubes.

"To prevent precipitation of minerals and return them to solution if precipitated, cider vinegar and water at mealtimes is the best answer." - Dr. D. C. Jarvis, *Arthritis & Folk Medicine*.

Dr. Jarvis claimed that ACV dissolves calcium deposits from the

---

[14] The sap from sugar maple trees boils in sugar-house kettles.

The Cure for Arthritis

joints and tissues of the body better than any other treatment. Other nutritional doctors, including Dr. Allen E. Banik, agree that apple cider vinegar is the best treatment for removing calcium deposits from the joints and tissues of the body.

Dr. Allen E. Banik:

"Apple cider vinegar is a tremendous solvent. Along with distilled water, you have an unbeatable team. Add a tablespoon or two of raw apple cider vinegar to a gallon of distilled water to give it flavor, and you have a drink fit for the gods. Vinegar removes water spots from the windows, which proves what an excellent solvent it is." - Dr. Allen E. Banik, *The Choice is Clear*.

Dr. Jarvis used the same ACV treatment for rheumatoid arthritis, osteoarthritis, gout and bursitis. Together with other nutritional doctors, such as Robert Morse and N. W. Walker, Dr. Jarvis did not differentiate between these diseases but considered them all to be various manifestations of arthritis. All of them have been successfully treated by the cider drink.

It is said that Cleopatra (c. 50 BC) dissolved precious pearls in natural vinegar. Pearls are made of calcium carbonate.

One of Dr. Jarvis' patients had extensive tartar deposits caked on his lower teeth. Within ten weeks of using only a teaspoon of ACV in a glass of water at each meal, the plaque totally disappeared.

Not all vinegars are alike. Most of the vinegars you buy in the salad dressing aisle at the supermarket are either distilled white vinegar, wine vinegar or balsamic vinegar. which are pasteurized food products. Pasteurization destroys the enzymes in the foods and decreases their nutrient content, whereas raw (unpasteurized) apple cider vinegar is rich in enzymes and nutrients.

The Cure for Arthritis

Apple cider vinegar is made by fermenting crushed apples, which also makes it different from other vinegars which are made by fermenting alcohol. ACV has the highest pH of any vinegar, 3.3 to 3.5. pH is a term used in chemistry for the amount of acidity or alkalinity of an aqueous solution. The pH scale runs from 0 to 14, with a pH of 7 being neutral, a pH of less than 7 being acidic, and a pH greater than 7 being alkaline. Other vinegars have a pH of around 2.4, making then more acidic. (pH is a logarithmic scale).

Nutritionists contend that vinegars other than ACV are harmful to the body since they contain only the destructive acetic acid. ACV has acetic acid and malic acid, an acid found in many fruits such as apricots, blackberries, blueberries, cherries, grapes, peaches, pears and plums, as well as apples, which has a number of health benefits, including combining with alkaline compounds and minerals in the body to produce energy, and aiding digestion.

Dr. N.W. Walker in his book *Fresh Vegetable and Fruit Juices*, states that apple cider vinegar contains malic acid, which is absent in white distilled and wine vinegars. Malic acid is beneficial to the body. All vinegars, including apple cider vinegar, are acidic, but as explained in his book, diluted apple cider vinegar is alkalizing to the body. In addition, malic acid can be stored in the body as glycogen for future use, and is known to promote healthy blood vessels, veins and arteries, and aid in coagulating the blood in establishing a normal menstrual flow.

As explained in Victoria Boutenko's book, *Green for Life*, hydrochloric acid (HCl) production in the stomach decreases after age 40. A low stomach acid condition is blamed for various nutritional deficiencies due to the inability of the body to adequately digest foods and absorb nutrients. It is also blamed for the greying of hair. Nutritional experts claim that

The Cure for Arthritis

supplementing the diet with apple cider vinegar helps to restore stomach acid to its proper levels.

Raw, unpasteurized apple cider vinegar contains the "mother", which is a murky substance found at the bottom of the bottle. The mother is rich in enzymes, pectin (the soluble fiber found naturally in apples), and organic minerals including magnesium, phosphorus, calcium and potassium. There is some evidence that the malic acid in apple cider vinegar helps to release iron from foods so that it can be better utilized by the body, and that the high potassium content of ACV helps to restore mineral balance to the body.

One of the benefits of ACV and honey is that it promotes sounder sleeps. Just a few teaspoons of apple cider vinegar and honey in a glass of water taken in the late afternoon or early evening can produce sounder sleep for the night.

It is noted that the Arthritis Foundation has included ACV on their list of food *myths* about arthritis. Its website claims that there is not enough evidence to suggest that ACV works to heal arthritis. However, this claim is not surprising when we learn that the Foundation receives much of its funding from the drug companies. Dr. Norman Childers tells us so in his book, *Arthritis - Childers' Diet That Stops It!*

Margaret Hills of Britain used ACV in her clinic to treat arthritis. As discussed in other chapters of this book, she believed that hard acid deposits are formed in the joints of the body by eating high acid foods, such as meat and dairy products, which are also high protein foods, and that these deposits are dissolved when diluted ACV is taken daily as part of a nutritional diet.

ACV has been used successfully to treat other health disorders besides arthritis, including candida, gum disease, chronic fatigue and high blood pressure. Margaret Hills noted that diluted ACV eliminated high blood pressure in many of her patients.

"Many arthritics suffer from high blood pressure, angina, or some form of circulatory disease. The taking of cider vinegar can be most beneficial in this case, as it is known to be a blood normalizer. If the blood pressure is to high, cider vinegar will help bring it down to normal, and if it is too low, it will raise it accordingly." - Margaret Hills, *Treating Arthritis: The Drug-Free Way.*

The Margaret Hills treatment for arthritis may best be summarized as follows. Eat a nutritional, low-acid diet and drink well-diluted apple cider vinegar. We should remember that Mrs. Hills cured herself of *both* osteoarthritis and rheumatoid arthritis by this treatment.

My experiences with the cure are given in the chapter on "My Story."

More About Honey

Honey is made by bees from the nectar of flowers and plants that bees visit when pollenating them. Raw honey contains many minerals, amino acids and enzymes.

Most of the honey consumed today is refined honey which is pasteurized so its enzymes have been destroyed. If the label does not say "raw," then it is refined and processed honey.

Dr. Jarvis in his book, *Arthritis and Folk Medicine*, states that the nutritional value of foods is improved by the ability of honey to extract from the foods what the body needs. He also states that it has been the experience of generations of Vermonters that beekeepers do not have kidney trouble and do not develop cancer or paralysis.

Organic, raw, unfiltered honey has not been adulterated in any way and is the best honey to eat for health benefits. It may be purchased from whole food stores or on the Web.

So, there you have it, a natural food product that dissolves unwanted calcium and possibly other inorganic minerals from the joints and tissues of the body. Cider vinegar and honey may be one of the best treatments for arthritis ever discovered.

Distilled Water

Regular water, such as faucet water and most bottled waters, comes from municipal water supplies and contains inorganic minerals, such as calcium. This is especially true if you live in areas of the country that have large deposits of limestone. As explained above, we should minimize our intake of inorganic minerals, including calcium. Furthermore, as explained in the next chapter, calcification of the joints is one of the causes of arthritis.

In the book, *Water, The Shocking Truth That Can Save Your Life*, Paul C. Bragg explains how growing up on a farm in Virginia exposed him to many people who had arthritis. Their water came from wells and had high concentrations of calcium carbonate and other inorganic minerals from the limestone deposits in the area. His grandfather died in his mid-sixties. The autopsy revealed that his arteries had turned to stone. A worker on the farm developed arthritis in her hands, wrists, elbows, hips, knees and ankles. She was tormented day and night by the pains and never reached 65. From such experiences, Bragg went on to formulate his Bragg Healthy Lifestyle which includes drinking plenty of distilled water. He lived arthritis-free to age 81.

The Cure for Arthritis

"Let us state emphatically that, in our opinion, the misery of arthritis is caused by ingestion of hard water saturated with inorganic minerals and toxins and an unhealthy diet. These factors combined with inactivity can form acid crystals in the movable joints. Ill health is the result of a combination of unnatural living habits! Every effect must have a cause. There is a reason why things happen in the body. It is failure to live Mother Nature's healthy lifestyle that is the cause of human miseries." - Paul C. Bragg, *Water, The Shocking Truth That Can Save Your Life*.

Distilled water is regular, hard water that has been boiled and steam condensed. Distillation is the most effective method of purifying water. The minerals stay behind because they are not volatile, and the condensed steam is pure of minerals, bacteria, viruses and physical impurities.

"There is only one way you can purify your body and help to eliminate your chronic aging diseases, and that is through the miracle of distilled water." - Dr. Allen E. Banik, *The Choice is Clear*.

Many nutritionists believe that drinking distilled water is beneficial to human health. Contrary to popular belief/misconception, distilled water does not leach out minerals that have become part of the body's cells. What it can do is leach out excess minerals that are deposited in the joints and tissues of the body, which are minerals the body could not properly utilize. This fact has particular importance for sufferers of arthritis.

Again, Dr. Banik:

"According to medical science, there is no sure cure for arthritis. Arthritis is partially caused by mineral deposits in the joints. X-rays will show the mineral deposits very clearly. These deposits crystalize to irritate the joints as they move, causing severe pain and swelling. Since the average person drinks up to 450 glasses of mineral solids found in hard water during a lifespan, it is logical to assume that these inorganic minerals were slowly deposited in the joints through the years, causing the arthritis. Distilled water, in turn, dissolves these mineral deposits." - Dr. Allen E. Banik, *The Choice is Clear.*

For more information about the benefits of drinking distilled water, see the chapter on "Distilled Water." For my experiences with distilled water, see the chapter on "My Story."

Niacin (Vitamin B3) Therapy

Improvement in the range of joint movement for people with arthritis has been experienced with relatively large doses of niacin.

Dr. William Kaufman, a major proponent of the use of niacin in reversing the symptoms of arthritis, claimed that niacin could reduce the joint swelling that is caused by arthritis. He developed instruments and a system for measuring joint mobility before and during the therapy, and photographed before and after arthritic conditions of his patients. Most of his work on vitamin therapy was done in the 1940s.

In the book, *Niacin, The Real Story*, by Abram Hoffer, Andrew W. Saul and Harold D. Foster, an entire chapter is devoted to Kaufman's pioneering work with niacinamide, which is a non-flush type of niacin.

"It has been demonstrated that when people supplement their good or excellent diets with adequate amounts of niacinamide, there is, in time, measurable improvement in ranges of joint movement, regardless of the patient's age. In general, the extent of recovery from joint dysfunction of any given degree of severity

depends largely on the duration of adequate niacinamide therapy."
- William Kaufman, M.D, PhD, *Niacin, The Real Story.*

In the above excerpt, it is noted that Dr. Kaufman indicates that only when the diet has been changed to a healthy diet should the treatment be taken.

There are three types of niacin: regular niacin, niacinamide and inositol hexaniacinate. Of the three, only regular niacin causes what is known as the niacin flush, which is an uncomfortable side effect experienced by people taking it.

My experiences with niacin are described in the chapter on "My Story."

A notable achievement of vitamin therapy in general is that some human diseases, such as pellagra, have been virtually wiped out by the compulsory enrichment of bread with thiamin, niacin, riboflavin and iron, which began in the US in 1943.

Sensitivities to Certain Foods

Sensitivities to certain foods, such as nightshade vegetables, have been known to cause the symptoms of arthritis in many people. In recent times, a proponent of curing arthritis by eliminating nightshades from the diet has been Dr. Norman F. Childers, who did most of his work between 1960 and 1980, and cured himself of osteoarthritis. He died at the age of 100 in 2011.

Nightshades are plants that contain solanine and/or nicotine, chemicals that for hundreds of years have been known to cause arthritis in grazing animals. Nightshade vegetables contain similar glycoalkaloids as found in the tobacco plant. Nightshade vegetables include tomatoes, eggplant, potatoes (white, yellow and red, but not sweet potatoes[15]), and peppers, such as chili peppers, paprika and lesser known plant foods, but does not include black or white pepper.[16]

In addition, several condiments and other common food items contain nightshade vegetables as ingredients, such as hot salsa, ketchup and marinara sauce.
Dr. Childers' book, *Arthritis - Childers' Diet That Stops It!*, includes testimonies of individuals who were completely cured of their arthritis by avoiding nightshade vegetables and condiments from their diets.

My experiences with a no-nightshades diet are described in the chapter on "My Story."

Fasting

Fasting is purposely depriving the body of food, particularly food that is difficult to digest. Freshly-squeezed fruit juices may be allowed on fasts since they are easily digested in less than about 30 minutes and do not tax the enzyme reserves of the body.

The cure for arthritis does not require fasting since the cure can be achieved without it. However, fasting signifies, and in the practice of fasting is found, almost all of the health principles that are elucidated in this book. Therefore, the reader should determine if fasting should be practiced in their health regimen for arthritis based on the severity of their condition and the information contained in this book about the importance of fasting in achieving optimal health.

---

[15] Sweet potatoes are not of the same plant family as the common white, yellow or red potatoes.
[16] Black and white pepper are derived from peppercorns, which are not in the nightshade family

The Cure for Arthritis

The evidence amassed on fasting cures for arthritis, as well as for other diseases, points not only to the importance of depriving the body of foods that bring on health problems and eating foods that promote healing and the restoration of health, but also to the importance of eating less food. Many nutritional experts contend that in order to achieve optimum health some form of fasting, even if it is just eating less during meals, should be practiced regularly.

Fasting is drugless therapy. It can overcome practically any ailment common to humankind. The clinical evidence for this is very compelling, as we will see.

"Take food away from a sick man's stomach and you have begun, not to starve the sick man, but the disease." - George F. Pentecost.

Fasting may be new to the reader. I did not start fasting until in my later years, and only after I learned from books about how important fasting is for attaining optimum health. It may just be that the practice of fasting is, for most people, and particularly for most people in this country, an unknown quantity. How many people do you know who fast? Have you ever fasted? Have you ever skipped at least three meals in a row, and on purpose?

Many people relate fasting to a religious rite, such as Lent or Ramadan. However, fasting is one of the oldest customs of which there is any record. It has been practiced for thousands of years in many cultures as an essential part of healing whatever is wrong with the body. Fasting is referenced many times in both the Old and New Testaments of the Bible.

The purpose of fasting is to relieve the body of the great expenditure of energy that is required to digest foods. Digestion is considered by nutritionists to be the most energy-intensive process carried out in the human body. It is said that the stomach

The Cure for Arthritis

is the most over-worked organ because it never gets a break, except maybe at nights. In Western society, most of us are munching on something all of the time. Is there ever a time when your stomach is not busy digesting foods?

In the past 150 years, the scientific and clinical data obtained from fasting performed in the health clinics and sanatoriums of Europe and the US tell us what occurs in the body during a fast and how fasting enables the body to heal itself of diseases.

Dr. Ann Wigmore and others tell us that when animals get sick they instinctively abstain from all food. Can this be said about us? To a great extent, it cannot. Most people keep eating when they are sick on the mistaken belief that nourishment is needed for them to get well. Only rarely, such as in cases of acute fever, do we lose our appetite for food. Most doctors prescribe nourishment for those who are sick in hospitals, or who are otherwise under their care, and many patients force themselves to eat when the wisest thing to do would be to abstain from all food. It appears that in this context, animals are wiser than humans.

"Fasting works by self-digestion. During a fast your body intuitively will decompose and burn only the substances and tissues that are damaged, diseased or unneeded, such as abscesses, tumors, excess fat deposits, excess water and congestive wastes. Even a short fast (1 to 3 days) will accelerate elimination from your liver, kidneys, lungs, bloodstream and skin. Sometimes you will experience dramatic changes (cleansing and healing crisis) as accumulated wastes are expelled. With your first fasts you may temporarily have cleansing headaches, fatigue, body odor, breath coated tongue, mouth sores and even diarrhea as your body is cleaning house. Please be patient with your body!" - Paul C. and Patricia Bragg, *Water, The Shocking Truth That Can Save Your Life,*

The Cure for Arthritis

Naturopathic healers and fasting professionals, including those who work in the renowned health clinics of Norway, Sweden and Germany, such as the Buchinger-Wilhelmi fasting clinic in Germany, are keenly aware of how fasting can cure diseases. They witness daily the amazing results brought about by fasting cures, and consider fasting to be the most important curative measure in disease treatment.

Many health advocates and raw foodists regularly fast for days at a time, including Professor Spira (his book is listed in the Bibliography).

Clinical Evidence on Fasting Cures

A vast amount of clinical evidence has been obtained on fasting cures. It has resulted in thousands of publications attesting to the amazing power of fasting in enabling the body to heal itself of diseases and other health issues. They include case histories of "miraculous" cures, some of which are without precedent.

The results of a small sampling of the clinical evidence of fasting cures are given below. The first two are taken from Arnold Paul De Vries' book, *Therapeutic Fasting*.

1. 715 cases of disease were treated by fasting in Dr. James McEachen's sanatorium. The diseases included heart disease, cancer, high blood pressure, kidney disease, ulcers, colitis, arthritis and multiple sclerosis. Remedied or greatly improved by fasting were 29 of 33 cases of heart disease, 20 of 23 cases of ulcers, 3 of 4 cases of multiple sclerosis, 36 of 41 cases of kidney disease, 77 of 88 cases of colitis, 39 of 47 cases of arthritis and all of the cancer and high blood pressure cases.

2. 155 cases of disease, including a similar spectrum of diseases as indicated above, were treated through fasting by Dr. William L Esser. 113 cases experienced complete recovery, 31 experienced partial recovery, and the remaining 12 cases experienced no benefit. The percentage of improved or remedied cases was 92.3%.

3. Edward Hooker Dewey, M.D. in his books, *The True Science of Living* and *The No-Breakfast Plan and the Fasting Cure*, recounts how hundreds of patients, many of whom had the most distressing diseases, were completely cured of their diseases by fasting.

4. Hereward Carrington in his book, *Vitality, Fasting and Nutrition*, gives many testimonies of healing from people who were completely cured of their diseases, including paralysis and deafness.

5. Upton Sinclair in his book, *The Fasting Cure*, gives many testimonies of healing from people who were completely cured of their diseases.

The evidence gained from studies such as these indicates that fasting is the most effective method of remedying any disease or other ill-health condition. Can mainstream medicine make such claims? Does it have similar success rates in its attempts at curing the same diseases? Do the success rates of conventional medical doctors and hospitals even approach those that are obtained from fasting? Mainstream medical treatments, including surgery, chemotherapy and drugs, cannot match or even come close to the efficacy of fasting in curing diseases.

Those who have seen how fasting can cure diseases say:

"Fasting is the most efficient means of correcting any disease." - Dr. Adolph Mayer.

"Fasting is like surgery without a lancet. It cuts away the superfluous and spares what is healthy." - Erwin Hof.

"Arthritis and related diseases are usually speedily remedied by fasting, with gradual disappearance of the severe pains and swelling and the complete or partial absorption of the deformity by autolysis, providing complete ossification of the joint is not present. Fasts of one to four weeks usually alleviate arthritis, with longer fasts being employed if deformities are present." - Arnold Paul De Vries, *Therapeutic Fasting*.

"The fast is to me the key to eternal youth, the secret of perfect and permanent health. I would not take anything in all the world for my knowledge of it. It is Nature's safety valve, an automatic protection system against disease." - Upton Sinclair, *The Fasting Cure*.

For more details, the reader is referred to the books in the Bibliography by Arnold Ehret, Paavo O. Airola, Herbert M. Shelton, Arnold Paul De Vries, Edward Hooker Dewey, Upton Sinclair, Paul C. and Patricia Bragg, and Kristine Nolfi.

Unlike conventional medical methods of disease treatment that suppress one symptom only to create others, fasting helps all the organs and tissues of the body equally, with no part being helped more than another, and no part being helped at the expense of another. Fasting works on the entire body.

Whenever a cure for a disease is effected and the hand of the destroyer is stayed, it should be headline news in the media and big news in the medical profession, even if it is accomplished outside the accepted norms and teachings of conventional medicine. But how are fasting cures treated by the media or looked upon by mainstream medicine? With disdain and nonacceptance. Why? Because fasting cures do not conform to the modus operandi of the mainstream medical profession.

Were mainstream medicine, in its efforts to cure diseases, to even come close to the success rates of fasting cures, it would be such a boon to civilization that it would likely eclipse all of the technological breakthroughs that have occurred in the last 120 years.

T. Colin Campbell and Howard Jacobson, in their book *Whole: Rethinking the Science of Nutrition,* describe in detail the numerous ways in which the medical industry has sacrificed health and the curing of disease for ever-increasing profits.

"Health information is controlled, and has been for a long time, by interests that are not in alignment with the common good – industries that care much more about their profit than our health. And those industries feel deeply threatened by the possibility of mass adoption of a plant-based diet." - T. Colin Campbell and Howard Jacobson, *Whole: Rethinking the Science of Nutrition.*

Imagine, if you will, that the next time you visited a doctor, he or she advised you not to take standard medical treatments, such as medication, for your ailment, but to perform a fast. Imagine what a shock that would be to your sensibilities. But don't worry, based on the past two hundred years of standard medical practice, it is not likely to happen in our lifetime.

Despite the prejudice that mainstream medicine seems to have against fasting cures in preference to their own methods of disease treatment, the facts continue to speak for themselves.

The Cure for Arthritis

Fasting allows the body to remove the causes of an ill-health condition rather than mask its symptoms. Healing is accomplished naturally when the internal energy required for digestion is turned off and made available for bodily healing and regeneration.

The body is the greatest healing machine ever. It only requires the right conditions to accomplish what it alone knows how to do.

When a person fasts, food intake is stopped and the entire digestive system, including all the major organs of the body, takes a very needed physiological rest. It is this rest that allows the body to focus more on self-cleansing and on whatever needs to be healed.

During a fast, the body is amply supplied with food from within, from its stored food reserves. The food reserves of the body are so vast that death by starvation does not occur in a matter of days, but months, which is typically much longer than the average time required for healing and recovery from a fasting cure.

Francoise Wilhelmi de Toledo, in her book, *Therapeutic Fasting: The Buchinger Amplius Method*, states that a person can live on body fat for up to 40 days without suffering any harm.

There are numerous references to fasting in the Bible. Two of the most memorable fasts are those of Moses and Jesus. Both fasts were for 40 days and 40 nights (i.e., 40 complete days). Moses's fast was before he received the Ten Commandments. Jesus' fast was before He began His ministry.

Many people look on these fasts as curiosities rather than facts. Some attribute them to the divine power that both Moses and Jesus had, which, of course, is the same as saying that their fasts were miracles which would not be possible for normal people under normal circumstances.

But saying that long duration fasts were, or are, miracles is refuted by the clinical evidence we have of people fasting for very long periods of time. Arnold Ehret, for example, fasted for 49 days, which was the world's record at the time. Dr. Kristine Nolfi and Dr. Wilhelmi de Toledo in their books tell us that fasts of more than 60 days have been performed in their clinics to cure diseases.

The Reluctance to Fast

In my opinion, although I hope I am wrong, fasting will never be a popular cure for disease or any other health disorder because it involves too much self-denial. In addition, a knowledge of fasting is required to go forward with the practice.

Many people today do not want to go without food for any length of time, much less for the time it takes to do a legitimate fast. I believe it has much to do with our eating habits. But there's also the hubris connected with eating in this country, the pride of having a surfeit of food. We have more food than our population needs, or can use, and in such variety and availability that it is the envy of the world. So, why pass up the opportunity to indulge while you can? It speaks of the "eat, drink and be merry, for tomorrow we die" attitude exposed in the Bible. It speaks of the dog-eat-dog, haves-and-haves-not world in which we live. It also suggests many of the attitudes that were prevalent in the ancient Roman Empire before its decline and fall.

Another reason that people do not want to fast is because they do not want to miss out on the pleasures of eating, and, in particular, eating foods that stimulate the pleasure centers of the brain, such as sugary foods, meat and dairy products, and salty, oily and/or greasy foods.

But regardless of how much we may like to eat, the fact remains that eating is one of the major causes of pain and suffering in the world. By consuming foods that are bad for us, and maintaining improper eating habits, we reap the consequences of ill-health and disease. However, if we give up harmful pacifiers for the brain and palate, and focus on foods that truly nourish us, foods that are needed by the body for cellular reconstruction and health, and do not contain toxins that end up being stored in the body's tissues and joints, then these harmful consequences can be avoided. Not only that, but a daily diet of raw fruits and vegetables sharpens the taste buds so flavors we never knew existed before can be enjoyed.

Fasting should be more acceptable and easier for those who are already accustomed to self-denial, repentance and humility.

Other Considerations

Wallace D. Wattles in his book, *Health Through New Thought and Fasting*, states that all overeating comes from the false belief that strength is gained by eating food.

Conventional wisdom and the claims of the food industry insist that we need high protein food to be strong and heathy. But this appears to be very misleading and wrong. As explained elsewhere in this book, raw plant foods, which are not high protein foods, provide all the protein needed for a healthy, active life. Also, the protein in plant foods is not the hard to digest protein of meat and dairy products. As discussed in the chapter on "The Causes of Arthritis," animal protein is complex protein that must be broken down before it can be assimilated by the body. The

The Cure for Arthritis

breaking down process results in the generation of an excessive amount of uric acid, which is known to cause uric acid crystals to form in the body that cause kidney stones and gout.

Wattles challenges us to prove conventional wisdom wrong by eating natural plant foods exclusively, cutting out one meal a day, and taking 24-36-hour fasts once a week for 4-5 months.

I followed Mr. Wattles' advice and can testify that it makes a big difference in the energy levels and feelings of well-being that I have. I skip breakfasts entirely, never eating anything until later in the mornings.

Clinical studies on fasting prove that a person does not become weaker by fasting, but that the strength of the body increases without foods, especially high protein foods. This is the opposite of what we have been led to expect, but it is true.

"Contrary to popular belief, you don't get weakened or depleted by fasting. On the contrary, fasting will strengthen the body in many ways. The stomach and digestive tract will receive a rest and will be strengthened by fasting." - Paavo O. Airola, N.D., *There is a Cure for Arthritis*.

Fasts longer than a week are typically recommended to allow the body to cure diseases. In general, the worse the disease or health condition, the longer the fast should be to correct the situation.

Note: For fasts over a week long, it is recommended, for possible medical complications, that the supervision of a physician or fasting professional be obtained.

My experiences with fasting are described in the chapter on "My Story."

The Efficacy of Alternative Medicine Treatments

Naturopathic healing has different degrees of success on different people. But there are reasons for this. The level of commitment that a person has when taking a natural cure is extremely important. If the initial desire to be completely healed wanes after a short while, if the person quits the cure before it has a chance to work, or no longer has the time available for seeing the cure through to completion, then the degree of success of the cure will vary accordingly. But that should not dissuade anyone from taking natural treatments for health disorders. A cure that works for some people may very well work for you too.

Not only that, but when a cure follows proven principles of health, and works in ways that address the underlying causes of the disease or health disorder that allow the body to heal itself, it is likely to produce the results that are expected.

What I consider to be a significant advantage of natural cures over other treatments for arthritis, such as standard medical treatments, is that they allow a person to make body-specific adjustments to suit their own condition. For example, instead of being given a prescription and told that you must not reduce or exceed the dosage, or the time period over which the dosage must be taken, alternative medicine treatments essentially allow you to make up your own prescriptions, and change them whenever you like as the body gives you feedback on the efficacy of the cure. This is especially true for cures that involve proper diet, since people have slightly different nutritional requirements.

Because we are part of Nature, we find that natural cures work the best for us. As seen in the next chapter, natural cures address the underlying causes of arthritis.

Chapter Summary

As discussed in this chapter, successful cures for arthritis and other diseases have been achieved through alternative medicine treatments and by a combination of them. Many books describe these cures, including those that are referenced in this book by Carrington, Sinclair and Childers. They are worth reading just for the testimonies they contain of individuals who were cured of their condition by these treatments.

Such successes bear out what Hippocrates said years ago, "Natural forces within us are the true healers of disease."

The Causes of Arthritis

It is the firm contention of many nutritionists and nutrition-minded medical doctors, many of whom are referenced in this book, that the causes of arthritis are not what mainstream medicine says they are, such as wear and tear, or degeneration, of the joints, joint misalignments and accidents and injuries. None of these causes have led to a cure, which strongly suggests that they are not the underlying causes of the disease at all, but only contributing causes or factors that can localize the disease to certain parts of the body. Before arthritis can be cured, the underlying causes of the disease must be understood.

Much of what has already been discussed in this book has provided important clues as to what causes arthritis. This chapter describes in detail what these causes are.

High on the list of what causes arthritis is poor nutrition. This should come as no surprise to anyone who has seen the ill-effects that commonly consumed foods and drinks have on people. As stated in the last chapter, in food lies nearly all of the causes of disease and imperfect health of any kind. Consequently, all healing must place emphasis on proper nutrition.

Nutritional Deficiency

Nutritional deficiency is rampant in this country, despite the abundance and availability of the foods that we have. Much of this deficiency is the result of the ubiquitous use of food refining and processing techniques, but it is also caused by farming practices, including the shift from small-scale farming to large-scale farming that has taken place in the last 60 years, topsoil mineral deficiency, the use of synthetic fertilizers on crops, and the proliferation of Concentrated Animal Feeding Operations (CAFOs) that keep springing up everywhere. The proliferation of these animal-factories has created the need for GMO crops, together with their deadly pesticides and herbicides. The result is that the nutritional value of foods in this country is no longer what it used to be.

The main contributor to the decrease in the nutritional value of foods is worldwide topsoil mineral deficiency. The topsoil in which plants are grown is now depleted of its minerals. Reports on the Internet cover recent losses of nutrients in crops. Only decades ago, the same crops were richer in vitamins and minerals. Meat and dairy products (animal products) are affected even worse. Animals consume the mineral deficient crops and become mineral deficient. Cooking animal products further depletes them of minerals and vitamins.

The mineral deficiency of the topsoil is being blamed on improper farm management practices resulting in ill-replenishment of the minerals back into the soil. The meteoric rise in food productivity and efficiency since the last century have not been balanced by a corresponding increase in the addition of nutrients back into the soil.

Nutritional deficiency occurs when the body does not absorb or get enough of the necessary amounts of nutrients it needs from foods. Nutrients include vitamins, minerals, proteins, carbohydrates, fats and water. They are essential for cellular growth and the maintenance of life. The body does not manufacture nutrients, but obtains them from the surrounding environment. We get most of our nutrients from foods.

On a whole plant food diet, there is no need for multivitamin /mineral supplements, since all the minerals and vitamins needed to support life are in raw plant foods in their proper organic form and undestroyed by heat. An example is the amount of organic calcium in collard greens. According to the USDA publication Nutritive Value of American Foods, just two-thirds cup of collard greens has 91% of the calcium in a cup of milk. Other plant foods having about the same amount of calcium are kelp and almonds.

A whole plant food diet also compensates for topsoil mineral deficiency since more plant foods are eaten on the diet. In addition, the diet includes sea vegetables, which are grown in the ocean -- a mineral-rich environment.

Nutritional deficiency is so widespread in this country and in the world today that it can be said to be the number one health problem in the world, even among people who supposedly eat a healthy, balanced diet. Ignorance of what constitutes a healthy diet can cause not only arthritis, but other diseases to take root in the human soil of the body.

The foods that are the best for health are those that have their vital nutrients and enzymes intact (the body requires nutrients, and enzymes to break down the nutrients, for foods to be assimilated in the body). All the minerals and vitamins needed to support life are in whole plant foods in their proper organic form and undestroyed by heat.

Acidity

Acidity is a blood condition mainly brought on by eating acid-forming foods, but drugs, caffeine and alcohol also create acidity in the body. According to leading nutritionists, acid-forming foods are responsible for many of the health issues and diseases that are prevalent in the world today, including diabetes and kidney failure.

The Cure for Arthritis

Common indicators of bodily acidity include headache, heartburn, and stomachache.

Refined grain and cereal products, refined sugar, meat products, including sausages and hot dogs of beef or pork, and pasteurized dairy products are widely eaten today. All leave behind a residue of toxic acids in the body. Modern refining techniques, including the use of high-temperature heat treatment and over-cooking, destroy the alkaline mineral salts found in natural foods that act to neutralize these acids.

If the acids go unchecked, they form hard acid deposits in the system. The soft tissues of the body, including those in the throat and anus, are the first affected. Eventually, the acids are deposited in the muscles, joints and ligaments of the body, which can cause arthritis and many other diseases such as bursitis, colitis and diverticulitis.

Patricia Bragg in her book, *The Miracle of Fasting*, explains how after years of eating meat and dairy products and man-made foods, toxic crystals can accumulate in the joints and press against nearby nerves to cause pain. The crystals can cause a wearing away of the cartilage and the synovial fluid membrane, which eventually leads to a wearing away of the bone surfaces themselves, an irreversible condition.

Cooked foods create acidity in the body, whereas uncooked (raw) plant foods alkalize the body. Acidity in the body also occurs when foods are combined incorrectly. Foods improperly combined inhibit digestion and cause discomforts such as stomachache, abdominal pain and fermentation and gas. More about this in the chapter on "Guidelines that Don't Work and Laws that Do."

Acid-forming foods include foods high in protein, such as eggs and beans as well as meat and dairy products. High protein foods cause the nutrients to stick together, which leads to cellular starvation and death. The foods also cause mucus production in the body, which is considered a forerunner of disease.

"People are becoming more and more acid. The public is not told this because the powers that be do not want people to know what is being done to them. In the last few decades, this fatal condition appears to be on the increase." - Rich Anderson, *Cleanse & Purify Thyself.*

Homeostasis, the tendency of the body to maintain itself in stable chemical equilibrium, is the bodily process that continually tries to balance or stabilize the body from an acidic condition to a normal alkaline condition. Obviously, the effectiveness of the body's ability at doing this is encumbered or enhanced by the foods that are eaten, and how they are eaten.

An acidic blood condition often results from a nutrient deficient diet, such as the standard American diet. If the diet is continued, the blood condition worsens to where the body's attempts at homeostasis are not sufficient in neutralizing the acids. Toxic acids the body cannot expel as waste in its on-going self-cleansing efforts are stored in the tissues and joints.

Vegetables, including leafy greens, carrots, cabbage, tomatoes, raw nuts, seeds and Superfoods[17], are alkalizing to the body, creating an alkaline blood condition that is conducive to healing and regeneration.

---

[17] David Wolfe in his book, Superfoods, defines them as plant foods with super high-density nutritional value. Examples of superfoods are hemp seed, maca and cacao beans.

The Cure for Arthritis

Of all the foods that there are for us to eat, most people eat refined and processed foods, such as fast foods, canned and jarred foods, packaged bread and grain products, such as cereals, sweet rolls and pastries, packaged meat products, including steaks, sausages, bacon, ham, hot dogs and hamburgers, and dairy products including milk, cream and cheese products.

Refined and processed foods have been heat treated (cooked) and almost always contain refined salt (table salt), refined and processed ingredients such as high fructose corn syrup (HFCS) and monosodium glutamate (MSG), and man-made flavors, colors and preservatives, none of which are natural products.

Americans eat more cooked food than any people on earth, and spend more money on doctor bills and healthcare than any people on earth. The fast food franchises, as well as other eating establishments, grill, fry, bake, steam-heat their foods, or use dehydrated foods that have already been refined and processed using these methods. It has been known for years that these methods destroy important food components such as enzymes, vitamins and other nutrients, and alter the chemical properties of the foods. Without sufficient nutrients in the diet, these foods leave behind the toxic acid residue that causes hard acid deposits in the joints.

In contrast, nutritionists tell us that our bodies are biologically suited for alkaline-forming foods, which are the fruits and vegetables found in nature. Since these foods neutralize acids that can cause disease, heartburn, upset stomach, indigestion, flatulence and other complications, we need to eat plenty of these foods.

Stress produces acidity in the body. High levels of stress have been linked to all kinds of physical and mental disorders. This acid-producer seems to have taken up permanent residence in our society.

"You must remove the obstructions and acidosis, if you don't, the cause remains as you have treated only the effect which can be swelling, pain or other symptoms. These are nothing more than natural defenses of the body in response to the cause. Detoxification is the only logical answer that will yield a lasting cure. Alkalization is the method by which detoxification starts. Alkalization neutralizes acidosis. Detoxification not only alkalizes the body, but also gives the body the added energy it needs to clean itself." - Robert Morse, N.D., *The Detox Miracle Sourcebook*.

The important subject of detoxification is discussed in the chapter on "How to Change the Situation."

Berg's Tables, in Appendix I, list what foods are "acid-forming" and "acid-binding." According to these tables, meat and grain products are the most acid-forming foods, whereas fruits and vegetables are the most acid-binding (alkalizing) foods.

"A person recovering or recovered from arthritis should always be careful with acid-forming foods: bread, cereals, animal proteins, cheese, etc. It is imperative to continue with the program of vital nutrition long after recovery if lasting results are to be expected." - Paavo O. Airola, N.D., *There is a Cure for Arthritis*.

Nutritionists tell us that if we ate nothing but raw fruits and vegetables, our blood would be alkaline most of the time, except for periods of undue stress or when other causes of blood acidity are introduced.

The chapter on "The Blood" describes how blood tests are used in medical diagnosis in assessing the acidity of the body.

The Cure for Arthritis

Margaret Hills, who lived in Britain during the 50s and 60s, proved to everyone's satisfaction that a diet of acid-producing foods causes arthritis, and that when these foods are avoided and alkaline-producing foods eaten in their place, arthritic patients lose their pains and inflammation and recover from the disease.

Many people are not aware of the damage being done to their joints and tissues because of the foods and drinks they consume. A victim of rheumatoid arthritis and osteoarthritis, Mrs. Hills cured herself of both types, and went on to open a clinic to cure numerous others by putting them on a low acid, nutritional diet.

Mrs. Hills' treatment for arthritis may best be summarized as follows. Eat a nutritional, low-acid diet, eliminating acid-forming foods from the diet, including grains and grain products and high protein foods, and decrease the excess acid state of the body by drinking well-diluted apple cider vinegar.

"The underlying cause of the chief forms of arthritis, osteoarthritis and rheumatoid arthritis, is excess acidity in the body. When acids collect between joints, the pain on movement can be likened to a vicious stabbing. Sometimes the joints get locked and may stiffen altogether, until there is very little movement or, indeed, none at all. In some cases, the joints make a grating sound. This is called crepitus, the unpleasant sound of the joints moving on those hard acid deposits." - Margaret Hills, *Treating Arthritis: The Drug-Free Way.*

To avoid hard acid deposits from forming in the joints and tissues of the body, we need to avoid or cut back on grain products, meat and dairy foods, fatty foods, refined and processed foods (canned, jarred, etc.), fast foods and restaurant foods, and other cooked foods, all of which contribute to bodily acidity.

The Cure for Arthritis

All pasteurized food products, including fruit juices from 100% concentrate, are cooked foods. For a detailed discussion about the dangers of cooked foods, see the chapter on "Dangers to Avoid."

It is no coincidence that urgent care centers in this country have become as numerous and widespread as fast-food restaurants.

"With proper diet and treatment, the acid deposits can be dissolved away, alleviating the pain and halting the condition." - Margaret Hills, *Treating Arthritis: The Drug-Free Way*.

Calcification (Mineralization) of the Joints

"Arthritis is caused by calcium deposits in the cartilage of the joints." – Dr. N. W. Walker, *Fresh Vegetables and Fruit Juices*.

Most Americans take some type of inorganic multivitamin/mineral supplement on a daily basis, and millions of people take calcium supplements to prevent or forestall osteoporosis. Billions of dollars are spent each year on multivitamin/mineral supplements.

Doctors often prescribe medication that is calcium carbonate based, which is an inorganic mineral compound. Calcium carbonate is the main ingredient in almost all antacids, and is found in some brands of aspirin. Some $2 billion is spent yearly in the US alone on antacids, and $10 billion worldwide, according articles to the Web.

However, calcium carbonate can cause stomach acid to increase above normal levels, resulting in what is known as acid rebound. Acid rebound is what causes heartburn and regurgitation. People with chronic stomach trouble or stomach ulcers are advised to switch to calcium citrate, an organic form of calcium derived from plant foods.

The Recommended Dietary Allowances (RDAs) for calcium were developed by the Food and Nutrition Board (FNB) and provided by the National Institutes for Health (NIH). They are listed below.

Recommended Dietary Allowances (RDAs) for Calcium

Age	Male	Female	Pregnant	Lactating
0–6 months	200 mg	200 mg		
7–12 months	260 mg	260 mg		
1–3 years	700 mg	700 mg		
4–8 years	1,000 mg	1,000 mg		
9–13 years	1,300 mg	1,300 mg		
14–18 years	1,300 mg	1,300 mg	1,300 mg	1,300 mg
19–50 years	1,000 mg	1,000 mg	1,000 mg	1,000 mg
51–70 years	1,000 mg	1,200 mg		
71+ years	1,200 mg	1,200 mg		

Many people in this country adhere to these guidelines by consuming food products high in calcium and by taking calcium supplements. Most people are taught from day one to drink milk and eat cheese to get enough calcium for strong bones and teeth. The threat of osteoporosis has only increased the motivation for consuming dairy products on a daily basis. According to the USDA, milk production has grown from approximately 1.4 billion pounds in 2008 to nearly 16.6 billion in 2018. It may be said that many of us have a phobia about not getting enough calcium.

Most people are not aware that the RDA guidelines are meant to be met by eating a variety of foods that are derived from *diverse* food groups, rather than from one food group, such as dairy, and that they are not meant to be met by supplementation or fortification.[18]

Nevertheless, according to a Harvard T.H. Chan School of Public Health article published on the Web,[19] RDAs were established based on short-term maximum-calcium-retention studies. Longer duration studies have since been performed that cast doubt on the value of consuming the large amounts of calcium that are currently recommended for adults in the RDAs. In particular, the studies indicated that high calcium intake does not decrease a person's risk for getting osteoporosis. The following excerpt is taken from the article:

"In the large Harvard studies of male health professionals and female nurses, individuals who drank one glass of milk (or less) per week were at no greater risk of breaking a hip or forearm than were those who drank two or more glasses per week. When researchers combined the data from the Harvard studies with other large prospective studies, they still found no association between calcium intake and fracture risk. Also, the combined results of randomized trials that compared calcium supplements with a placebo showed that calcium supplements did not protect against fractures of the hip or other bones. Moreover, there was some suggestion that calcium supplements taken without vitamin D might even increase the risk of hip fractures. A 2014 study also showed that higher milk consumption during teenage years was not associated with a lower risk of hip fracture in older adults."

Nutritional experts, such as those referenced in this book, believe

---

[18] National Research Council Subcommittee on the Tenth Edition of the Recommended Dietary Allowances, National Academies Press, published on an NCBI website.
[19] Article entitled, "Calcium: What's Best for Your Bones and Health?"

that inorganic minerals, including calcium, which are found not only in multivitamin/mineral supplements but in mineral-fortified foods, such as calcium-fortified orange juice and cereals, cannot be properly utilized by the body. And what is not purged from the body as waste ends up in the joints and tissues of the body.

Dr. Norman W. Walker, Dr. Bernard Jensen, Dr. Ann Wigmore, Paul and Patricia Bragg and others argue in their books (see Bibliography) that it is virtually impossible for the body to utilize inorganic minerals. The nutritionists also assert that inorganic minerals not eliminated by normal bodily processes get stored in the body's tissues and joints. They firmly believe that we should get all our minerals from plant foods.

"Inorganic minerals are not completely purged from the body by the kidneys and other body organs -- only a portion of them are. The rest accumulate in the body tissues and joints. Over time, this accumulation of inorganic minerals results in various degenerative diseases, including arthritis. This accumulation is also said to be the cause of a general enfeebled rigidity called "old age." – Dr. N. W. Walker, *Water Can Undermine Your Health*.

Calcium is an inorganic mineral found in rocks and soil. It is also found in refined and processed foods and drinks, in most of the multivitamin/mineral supplements that are on the market today, and in faucet, spring and bottle waters, almost all the waters that are commonly consumed, except for distilled water.

The calcium that is found in plant foods is organic calcium, the form that meets the body's cellular requirements. Organic calcium protects the heart, whereas the inorganic calcium, the kind found in supplements, is known to increase the risk for cardiovascular events, including heart attacks.[20] [21]

The 2016 John Hopkins Medicine article cited below reported that based on 10 years of medical tests on more than 2,700 people in a federally funded heart disease study, researchers concluded that taking calcium in the form of supplements may raise the risk of plaque buildup in arteries and heart damage, although a diet high in calcium-rich foods appears be protective. The coauthor of the report stated:

"There is clearly something different in how the body uses and responds to supplements versus intake through diet that makes it riskier." - John Anderson, Ph.D.

The days when milk cows roamed the pastures and got their calcium from grass are over. Today's milk cows do not go outside to graze. They seldom move out of their stalls or feedlots. Their urine and feces are removed mechanically. Their milk is removed by machines hooked up to their udders. They get their calcium and other nutrients from their feed, which, according to Web articles, is a specially formulated mix of grains, soy, silage and inorganic calcium in the form of calcite flour (calcium carbonate), aragonite (calcium carbonate), crushed bones, and other bits and pieces of slaughtered animals to maximize weight gain and therefore profits when the cows are no longer useful as money-making machines. Apparently, calcium from cow's milk is mostly inorganic calcium.

---

[20] 2016 John Hopkins Medicine report by Erin Michos, M.D., M.H.S. and John Anderson, Ph.D., entitled "Calcium Supplements May Damage the Heart."
[21] 2020 Mayo Clinic article on the Web, by Rekha Mankad, M.D., entitled "Calcium Supplements: A Risk Factor for Heart Attack?"

The Cure for Arthritis

If true, it would help explain the results of the Harvard T.H. Chan School of Public Health study cited above where researchers found no correlation between calcium intake and fracture risk, and also found that high calcium intake does not decrease a person's risk for getting osteoporosis. Both findings indicate that calcium from cow's milk is mostly inorganic calcium.

As stated in a 2015 Forks Over Knifes website article[22], the amount of calcium we ingest is not what we actually absorb. For example, a cup of milk contains about 300 mg of calcium, but only about 30% of it (90 mg) is absorbable in the body. In contrast, one cup of bok choy, 1-2 cups of kale, or 2 cups of broccoli is equivalent to the amount of calcium in a glass of milk because it is much easier absorbed.

David Wolfe in his book *Longevity Now*, explains how calcification of the joints causes the acute and chronic pains of arthritis. He states that "bad calcium" is calcium in the body that is harmful because of its insolubility and lack of electrons, and that the resulting calcification acts like sand in our biological gears and eventually results in clogging plaques that cause inflammation and pain.

All animals, including humans, need plants to obtain their minerals. Plants take up inorganic minerals from the soil and water and convert them into organic form, the form that is readily assimilated by the cells of the body. Ingesting foods and drinks that contain inorganic minerals, such as calcium, results in the deposition of those minerals in the joints and tissues of the body.

"Only a living plant's roots has the power to extract inorganic minerals from the earth and to transform them into useful organic

---

[22] Entitled, "Getting Clarity About Calcium," by Rosane Oliveira, DVM, PhD.

foods to nourish our miracle working bodies." - Paul C. and Patricia Bragg, *Water, The Shocking Truth That Can Save Your Life*.

Inorganic mineral supplements are also harmful to human health because they add to the toxic burden that the body must cope with. More is said about Inorganic mineral supplementation in the chapter on "My Story."

At the time of this writing, websites polled for information about the body's ability to utilize inorganic minerals loosely imply that the substances can be absorbed somewhat by the body, at least to some extent, which seems to be the consensus of mainstream medical professionals who prescribe inorganic mineral supplements, and supplements that have inorganic minerals in them, for their patients. But nutritional experts are telling us that these substances do us harm.

I am convinced that the key to improving health and well-being is self-education about foods and nutrition. Without this knowledge, and how ordinary diets bring about a large number of health disorders and diseases, including arthritis, we remain wholly ignorant of how to cure ourselves of arthritis and prevent other health disorders from taking root in the human soil of the body.

The knowledge that is needed about foods and nutrition is best obtained by reading books, and utilizing other learning tools such as the Web, to discover the truth about these subjects. But many of the vital truths about foods and nutrition are found only in books.

As mentioned in the chapter on "Arthritis 101," calcium and other mineral crystals are commonly found in synovial fluid samples of patients who are suffering from osteoarthritis, and it is believed that these crystals lessen or inhibit the cushion effect of the cartilage, which eventually causes the bones to rub against each other, resulting in the pain and inflammation of osteoarthritis.

Calcium crystals that are deposited in the joints and tissues of the body have been called Basic Calcium Phosphate (BCP) crystals. These crystals are insoluble at the body's pH levels, meaning that they cannot be purged from the body as wastes, but take up residence in the joints and tissues of the body.

A 2018 NCBI article on the Web,[23] reported that calcium pyrophosphate deposition (CPPD) disease is a type of arthritis, and is caused by the buildup of inorganic mineral crystals (for example, BCP crystals) in cartilage. It also stated that CPP crystals are commonly seen in spinal tissues, including inter-vertebral disks and spinal ligaments.

A 2019 NCBI article on the Web[24] states that acute arthritis attacks caused by BCP crystal deposition are common, and can cause the same inflammatory reactions in the joints and tissues of the body that monosodium urate crystals (uric acid crystals) cause in gout patients.

A 2018 NCBI article on the Web[25] reported that although the pathogenesis of CPPD disease is not fully understood, CPP crystal formation in the pericellular matrix of cartilage is the first step in the disease process.

---

[23] By Ann K. Rosenthal, M.D. and Lawrence M. Ryan, M.D., entitled, "Calcium Pyrophosphate Deposition Disease."
[24] By Dr, Shumaila M Iqbal, Internal Medicine, University at Buffalo / Sisters of Charity Hospital, et. al., entitled, "Updated Treatment for Calcium Pyrophosphate Deposition Disease: An Insight."
[25] By Ann K. Rosenthal, M.D. and Lawrence M. Ryan, M.D., entitled, "Calcium Pyrophosphate Deposition Disease."

The Cure for Arthritis

The information supports what nutritional experts have been telling us for years, that inorganic minerals that are not purged from the body as wastes infiltrate into the tissues and joints of the body, and, in time, their buildup interferes with the lubricating effect of the synovial fluid and reduces the spaces between the bones, resulting in the pains and inflammation of arthritis. Also, the bones may become locked (ankylosis) and enlarged (deformed) due to the buildup of these deposits.

In light of what nutritionists are telling us about what really causes arthritis, some of the causes that medical science attributes to arthritis, such as accidents, injuries, and the repetitive use of the joints, may break down the cartilage, or assist in breaking it down, but they do not in themselves cause mineral crystals to localize in these areas, Rather, it is what we put into our bodies, the foods and substances that we ingest, that are responsible for their formation.

To prevent calcification of the joints, nutritional experts recommend dietary change. In particular, they recommend avoiding dairy products and mineral supplementation.

Cartilage breakdown is also known to cause the bones to develop growths known as bone spurs. Bone spurs are, according to the many nutritionists, another result of ingesting foods and drinks that contain inorganic minerals, such as calcium. The body doesn't normally grow bone spurs, not if it is on a healthy diet. They are formed as a result of consuming foods and drinks that have these substances in them.

"Bone spurs and calcified formations are insoluble deposits that get into the tissues after consumption of water loaded with inorganic minerals, salt and uric acid, plus deposited toxic acid crystals from an incorrect diet high in acid. Meat, refined flour products, white bread, etc., coffee, sodas and sugary desserts are all high in acid content. This is the unhealthy dead-food diet that most people eat. This diet, combined with hard water, is why there are so many joint troubles resulting from acid deposits that create bone spurs and painful crystalized joints, etc." - Paul C. and Patricia Bragg, *Water, The Shocking Truth That Can Save Your Life.*

This section has shown that calcification (mineralization) of the joints is caused by inorganic calcium and other mineral deposition in the joints. The joints targeted for cartilage breakdown by these deposits may be determined by everyday joint usage, or by accident or injury, but these commonly considered causes of arthritis are not the underlying causes, but rather the foods and substances that are ingested which cannot be properly utilized by the body.

Toxicity

Toxicity is internal poisoning that is brought about by accumulated waste material in the body. According to nutritionists, it is the most common ill-health condition prevalent today. It is mainly the result of eating the wrong foods, such as animal-based foods that are baked or deep-fried in oils; starchy foods, including doughnuts, sweet rolls, pasta and bread; and other refined and processed, heat-treated foods, including canned, jarred and most packaged snack foods. Toxicity results from the morbid accumulation of toxins and food wastes in the organs and tissues of the body, and is similar to mucus buildup from eating mucus-producing foods.

"Disease is an effort of the body to eliminate waste, mucus and toxemias, and the system assists nature in the most perfect and natural way. Not the disease but the body is to be healed, it must be cleansed, freed from waste and foreign matter, from mucus and toxemias accumulated since childhood. You cannot buy health in a bottle, you cannot heal your body, that is, cleanse your system, in a few days, you must make "compensation" for the wrong you have done your body all during your life." - Arnold Ehret, *Mucusless Diet Healing System*.

According to nutritionist Robert Morse, mucus-forming foods are responsible for many types of inflammation in the body, such as the diseases that end in "itis", including bursitis and arthritis.

More about mucus-producing foods is discussed in the chapter on "Dangers to Avoid."

Secondary causes of toxicity in the body include the ingestion of chemical preservatives and man-made additives that are found in refined and processed foods, and the ingestion of pesticide residues on foods. Common medical practices also cause toxicity of the body, such as vaccinations and prescription drugs.

Poisons can also get into the body from the environment, from municipal drinking water, car exhaust fumes, cigarette smoke, and toxic chemicals that we become exposed to in the home and on the job. All contribute to the toxicity of the body. Some of these pollutants are carcinogenic or mutagenic. It seems very likely that exposure to these toxic substances will continue for some time to come in our society.

The result is that the body is made toxic by substances it ingests or is exposed to. The good news is that certain foods, such as green leafy vegetables, protect us from the harmful effects of carcinogens like no drug can. Chlorophyll in green plants detoxifies the liver and the bloodstream and neutralizes environmental pollutants. To receive this protection, all we need to do is include greens in our diet.

The Cure for Arthritis

Many people take inorganic substances in the form of multivitamin/mineral supplements on a daily basis. Billions of dollars are spent each year in America alone on these substances. Also, many take medication every day as prescribed by their doctors. As discussed previously, inorganic substances and drugs are not properly utilized by the body but are treated by the body as toxins. Many of them get stored in the body's tissues, including the cartilage collagen matrix in joints.

Some of the internal damage caused by toxic substances heals automatically. But when overloaded with toxins, the body cannot eliminate the poisons fast enough, which causes them to accumulate in the tissues. And that is when they can cause harm, such as weakening the immune system.

Commonly consumed foods, including meat, fish, eggs, and dairy products, contain substances that are toxic or otherwise harmful to the body, including carcinogens, hormones, dioxins, bacteria, and other contaminants that can accumulate in your body and remain there for years. Every year we hear of meat products contaminated with E. coli, listeria, campylobacter, or other dangerous bacteria that live in the intestinal tracts, flesh, and feces of animals.

Other commonly consumed food products contain substances that are known to be harmful to human health, including table salt, refined sugar, hydrogenated oils, preservatives, artificial colors and sweeteners, excitotoxins such as monosodium glutamate (MSG) and GMO (Genetically Modified Organism) food products such as High Fructose Corn Syrup (HFCS). All are unnatural substances produced by man-made processes.

Evidence from X-rays and autopsies of people with long histories of poor eating habits, such as eating a lot of cooked and starchy foods, reveals a plaster-like coating formed on the inner surfaces of the large intestine, or colon. This coating, or what many investigators call "plaque", prevents foods from being fully digested and assimilated, and often causes obstruction of the colon. In time, the coating builds up to where the intestines become mostly or even totally obstructed. A thorough discussion of intestinal obstruction, with sketches, is found in Dr. Norman W. Walker's book, *Become Younger.*

When the waste material in the large intestine, or colon, is not expelled at approximately the same rate as meals taken per day, then a state of constipation exists. It causes bodily toxicity. As explained in the chapter on "Arthritis 101," toxic substances can get into the cartilage and cause a gradual deterioration of its matrix, which leads to loss of cartilage function and the pains and inflammation of arthritis.

Constipation is a major cause of internal toxicity. It is worsened by the rapid growth of parasites that thrive and flourish in the rotting intestinal wastes. Stopped up wastes are a fertile breeding ground for many kinds of non-friendly parasites, including tapeworms which can cause many complications. A person may have a bowel movement once a day and think that everything is fine, but everything is not fine.

A bowel movement once a day is a sign of a serious health concern. It is a warning signal given by the body that something is wrong and should be corrected as soon as possible. Foods that are devoid of fiber, such as meats, dairy and white flour products, are known to cause constipation.

When in good health, one can expect to have as many bowel movements per day as meals taken per day. It is one of the gauges used for telling whether a person is in good health. Real freedom, no matter where you may be living, is constipated-free eliminations, probably the best comfort you can ever have.

Amazingly, constipation in this country is considered, like headache, heartburn, stomachache and fatigue, to be a normal condition of modern living. But like practically all sickness and disease, constipation does not occur by chance but is caused by the foods that are consumed.

The clogging up of the intestines caused by foods of ordinary diets causes intestinal bacteria to multiply inordinately which releases poisons into the blood stream. The state of constipation is the primary cause of illness and disease in the human body according to Dr. N. W. Walker, Professor Arnold Ehret, Dr. Ann Wigmore, Fred Hirsch, Karyn Calabrese, Professor Spira, and other nutritionists. They believe that disease symptoms are manifested as a result of this poisoning, and that they are signs the body gives when it attempts to eliminate the poisons. Malaise and fatigue are two typical signs of internal poisoning.

The blockage of wastes also hinders the absorption of nutrients in the body. Poor nutrient absorption leads to nutritional deficiency. If the food is nutrient-deficient in the first place, then even less nutrients are assimilated by the body.

Toxic wastes continue to build up until corrective action is taken. To avoid suffering from toxic waste health disorders, including arthritis, the most important thing we can do is to reduce or eliminate the intake of foods and supplements that cause toxic waste buildup, and eat whole plant foods instead. Antioxidant-rich foods are known to stop or even reverse toxic buildup. Whole plant foods are high in antioxidants that neutralize the poisons and help to flush them out of the system.

More information about how foods of ordinary diets cause intestinal clogging is included in the chapter on "Dangers to Avoid."

Uric Acid and Gout

Whenever we eat animal products, a particularly harmful acid is produced -- uric acid. Animal protein is complex protein that must be broken down before it can be assimilated by the body. The breaking down process results in the generation of an excessive amount of uric acid. Since the muscles of the body have an affinity for uric acid, it is initially deposited in the muscles. When the saturation point is reached and the uric acid is sent to the kidneys, uric acid crystals are formed which can cause kidney stones and gout.

In contrast to animal protein, plant protein does not cause uric acid production in the body. In addition, Dr. T. Colin Campbell states in his book, *The China Study*, that plant protein is the healthiest type of protein because it allows for slow but steady synthesis of the proteins. Eating a variety of greens ensures that we receive all the amino acids we need in our diets.

According to Norman W. Walker in his book, *Become Younger*, uric acid crystals can cause arthritis.

Summary of the Causes of Arthritis

A shown in this chapter, the causes of arthritis are:

1. Nutritional deficiency, caused by eating nutrient-deficient foods, which are the foods of common, or ordinary, diets.

2. Acidity, caused by eating acid-producing foods of ordinary diets. Acidity is also caused by constipation which is caused by eating foods of ordinary diets.

3. Calcification (mineralization) of the joints, caused by ingesting inorganic minerals that the body cannot properly utilize.

4. Toxicity, mainly caused by eating foods of ordinary diets and taking inorganic substances, such as those found in most multivitamin/mineral supplements. Constipation leads to toxicity of the body and results in blood poisoning by the toxins produced in the stopped-up waste material in the intestines. Constipation also hinders the absorption of nutrients in the body, which contributes to nutritional deficiency.

The above causes, which may all be said to be due to improper dietary practices, result in hard acid and mineral deposits forming in the joints and tissues of the body that cause the chronic symptoms of arthritis.

Gout, which is a type of arthritis, is caused by uric acid crystal deposition in the joints, which is, once again, caused by poor dietary practices.

Reflection

Fortunately, there are ways of dissolving hard acid and mineral deposits from the joints and tissues of the body into the bloodstream for their elimination through the normal elimination organs of the body, as will be seen in this book.

When confronted with a health issue, such as arthritis, we should do everything in our power to resolve it without resorting to doctors. As stated previously in the chapter on "The Importance of Alternative Medicine," when the cause and effect relationship between a health issue and what we are doing to ourselves becomes apparent to us, the best solution will then be known, as well as the proper steps that are needed to put it into effect.

How to Change the Situation

Anyone with a little persistence and willpower can change the way they are eating. True change always begins in the mind. Healthy eating habits are formed when we become convinced that dietary change is in our best interests.

However, many people believe that they are, and have been, living healthy lives, and in particular, they believe that they are eating healthy foods, even when they have health issues. But this is belied when the causes of disease and lesser health disorders are examined, as we have seen in previous chapters, and as we will also see in this chapter.

I grew up at the time when fast-food franchises were just starting out in this country. I was hooked on, and for years ate the foods of the Standard American Diet. But as I learned more and more about foods and nutrition, and saw all the ill effects that the diet had on myself and others, I began eating healthier foods.

In order to change the situation and cure arthritis, one must become convinced that they are doing themselves harm.

How Health Disorders are Linked to Unhealthy Diets

Increasing scientific evidence compiled every year links the top 10 leading causes of death, and the degenerative diseases so prevalent in the world today, to eating meat-based and dairy-based diets. These studies continue to show that people eating a plant-based diet have increased longevity and health compared to those eating a meat-based and/or dairy-based diet. Many books published in recent years provide the results of these clinical studies.

The Cure for Arthritis

The China Study, published in 2005, may be the most comprehensive study of human nutrition ever performed. The population, or group, that was used in the study was the entire population of China. Written by T. Colin Campbell, a professor of Nutritional Biochemistry at Cornell University, and his son Thomas M. Campbell II, a physician, the study proved that whole plant-based foods, not animal-based foods, are the most beneficial foods for people. The study showed that people eating a plant-based diet have increased longevity and health compared to those eating a meat-based and/or dairy-based diet.

How Not to Die, written by Dr. Michael Greger and published in 2015, confirmed the conclusions of *The China Study*, and provided additional research and study results that emphasized the importance of eating plenty of whole plant foods, such as fruits and vegetables, to prevent and even *reverse* the chronic diseases of the Western world, including cancer, diabetes, heart disease and brain diseases.

The hazards of eating animal-based foods, or animal products, are well known to most educated people. Eating animal products causes plaque formations in the arteries, which is known to cause hardening of the arteries, which can lead to heart disease and stroke. Harmful mutagens and carcinogens, such as acrylamide, HCAs, PAHs and AGEs, are formed when animal products are cooked (for more detail, see Victoria Boutenko's book, *12 Steps to Raw Foods*). Animal products can contain nitrates, chlorine and ammonia and are susceptible to hosting various forms of life-destroying bacteria.

Studies conducted on animals and people show that blood cholesterol levels increase when animal protein is eaten. Dr. Caldwell Esselstyn, Jr., in his book, *Prevent and Reverse Heart Disease,* says that anyone with high blood cholesterol levels is prone to heart disease. Animal-based foods contain cholesterol, whereas no plant foods contain cholesterol. Dr. Esselstyn changed his diet to a plant-based diet and strongly recommended his patients to do the same. Those who did were able to cleanse their coronary arteries of plaque formations, which means their arteries were no longer clogged, and Dr. Esselstyn proved this by way of coronary angiograms.

Dr. Esselstyn is now a leading advocate of raw plant foods. He is featured in the food documentary DVD, *Forks Over Knives*. Testimonies given in that DVD attest to the powers of raw plant foods to heal a number of leading chronic diseases, including heart disease and breast cancer.

In *Fruits and Farinacea -- The Proper Food of Man*, John Smith tells us that based on all accessible sources, our progenitors were frugivorous, i.e., fruit eaters. Both anthropological studies and studies of how the human body functions support this conclusion.

"Meat is not man's natural food, since he is not either a carnivorous or an omnivorous animal. Every argument drawn from comparative anatomy, from physiology, from chemistry, from experience, from observation, and, when rightly used, from common sense, all agree that man is not a meat-eating animal. He can never be as healthy under the prevailing "mixed" diet as he would if he were to follow the dictates of Nature and live on his natural food – fruits and nuts, eaten in their uncooked, primitive form. Every element the system needs can be shown to be present in these foods, in their proper proportion, while, being live foods instead of mere "dead ashes", which is all the cooking process leaves, they will be found to supply a degree of vital life and energy which no cooked foods ever supplied or could supply."
- Hereward Carrington, *Vitality, Fasting and Nutrition*.

The Cure for Arthritis

Human beings, in many key physiological ways, are not like other animals. We have hands with opposable thumbs, non-claw-like nails, teeth that are not suitable for tearing hide or flesh, or breaking bones, but rather for grinding plant foods, and long, not short, digestive tracts including 20-30 foot long intestines that are ideally suited for digesting fiber-rich foods like fruits, vegetables, nuts, seeds and grains.

David Wolfe in his book, *The Sunfood Diet Success System*, includes as Appendix A, an "Anatomy Chart" that identifies 17 physiological ways in which human beings are ideally suited for eating a plant-based diet. Websites also support this conclusion, as can be seen by searching on "are humans frugivores?"

These studies show that humans are naturally suited for picking, chewing and digesting plant-based foods. Chimpanzees, which are very similar to humans physiologically, subsist almost entirely on fruits and greens.

According to the Bible, the first people on earth lived to very great ages. Adam lived to 930 years   Methuselah lived 969 years. Prior to the Flood, the average human lifespan was about 900 years. However, immediately after the Flood, when animal food was permitted to be eaten, the average lifespan fell to about 400 years. Later, when Jacob, the father of the twelve tribes of Israel, lived, the average lifespan was only about 150 years.

Based on the latest worldwide statistics from WHO, the average human lifespan is currently 72 years.

We live in the age of information, and the Web/Internet is our most popular information source. While I consider the Web a very useful tool for learning about foods and nutrition, it should not be our only source for this information. Much of what is on websites is opinion-oriented or provided in support of commercial interests.

Opinions can run the gamut, and misrepresentation and conflicting information can be, and often times are, the result.

"As corrupting an influence as money is in medicine, it appears to be even worse in the field of nutrition, where it seems everyone has his or her own brand of snake oil supplement or wonder gadget. Dogmas are entrenched and data too often cherry picked to support preconceived notions." - Dr. Michael Greger, *How Not To Die*.

We cannot trust everything we read on the Web. But that being said, the Web should not be ignored as a learning tool in self-education about foods and nutrition. However, for those of us who are seeking answers to the really tough questions of today about foods and nutrition, books provide the answers. The books that are listed in the Bibliography are excellent resources that will aid anyone in their quest for a more thorough understanding of foods and nutrition, including the hottest health issues of today.

Books have the answers on how to gain optimum health, the Web does not. Books cannot be easily condensed into Web articles, and typically provide comprehensive coverage of the issues, or they refer to other books or studies that provide the information. In addition, books are typically written by competent and knowledgeable authors who provide good, proven advice.

it is our responsibility to take care of our bodies. It is not our doctor's, our spouse's, our friends' or the Government's. It is our responsibility. We should avoid foods that are harmful to health and eat foods that promote health and longevity. These are whole plant foods, replete with their life-giving properties.

Arthritis should not be looked on as an affliction brought on by fate or Providence, but something primarily, or perhaps even solely, brought on by an ignorance of the unalterable laws of nature, and most notably the laws governing foods and nutrition.

If fasting can cure almost all diseases of which the human race is susceptible, and it can, as seen in the chapter on "The Importance of Alternative Medicine," then what does that tell us about how diseases and other health disorders originate? Doesn't it clearly reveal that the principle cause of health disorders lies in the foods that are eaten? Does it not assuredly implicate improper diet as the main cause of many of our ailments?

"Disease stems from deficiencies and a lack of understanding of Mother Nature's laws of health, plus the unwillingness to accept the obligation to keep the precious temple – the body – in order. This is accomplished by keeping it clean and well-nourished. And, of course, providing necessary aids such as rest, relaxation, positive thinking and plenty of exercise through hard work." - Dr. Ann Wigmore, *Be Your Own Doctor*.

<u>The Plant-Based Diets</u>

For comparison purposes, the plant-based diets are as follows:

Vegetarian Diet – The vegetarian diet is a diet that consists mostly of plant foods. It minimizes meat and dairy products but can include some fish, and/or some dairy and poultry such as cheese and eggs. The emphasis of the vegetarian diet is on eating mainly plant foods but also cutting back on animal-based foods. Both cooked plant and animal-based foods are allowed on the vegetarian diet.

The Cure for Arthritis

Vegan Diet – The vegan diet is somewhat like the vegetarian diet but it goes further to exclude *all* animal-based foods, even fish, cheese and eggs. The vegan diet allows cooked plant foods to be eaten.

Raw Vegan Diet – The raw vegan diet is somewhat like the vegan diet in that it excludes all animal-based foods[26]. But it also excludes all cooked foods, which includes cooked plant foods.

A vegan or even a vegetarian diet can significantly reduce arthritic inflammation and pain. Even Web articles state this. However, a raw vegan diet, which goes further than both of these diets in excluding harmful foods, does it even better. Modern nutritionists, including those listed in the Bibliography, agree that the raw vegan diet, together with drinking distilled water and fasting, dissolves accumulated inorganic minerals and toxins that are deposited in the joints and tissues of the body better than any other health regimen.

Raw plant foods are foods as found in Nature. They enable the body to heal itself of diseases and attain optimum health. The reason they do this is because of the natural life force that is in these foods. This life force comes from the sun and is converted by plants into energy that humans and animals can utilize. When we eat raw (uncooked) fruits and vegetables, including green leafy

---

[26]Bee products are often contested as not being raw vegan food since they come from bees, which are animals. However, there are many nutritionists, among them Ann Wigmore, Norman W. Walker, Herbert M. Shelton and David Wolf, who advocate including bee products in the raw vegan diet. In my opinion, this issue is, in the overall picture of things, a minor point of contestability, especially when the health benefits of bee products are considered. In any case, each of us must decide how we stand on this issue. Like any other types of food, if bee products do not work for you, then they should be avoided

vegetables, we get the precious life force that God and Nature intended for us to receive.

Both the vegetarian and vegan diets restrict, or avoid, animal-based foods, which is to their credit. However, both allow cooked foods to be eaten, which is to their detriment, since cooked foods are harmful to human health.

The cooking of foods at home and in restaurants, and in the food factories that manufacture canned, bottled and jarred foods, reduces the food value of the foods by altering their chemical properties and destroying important food components, such as enzymes and nutrients, including vitamins and antioxidants.

If food is browned by heat treatment, such as by broiling, baking or deep frying, dangerous chemicals are created, such as advanced glycation end-products (AGEs), which have been known to cause diabetes and heart disease.

Almost every kind of food that comes in a sealed package (bag, box, can, jar, bottle, etc.) has been refined and processed, meaning, among other things, that it has been heat-treated. The enzymes in the foods have been destroyed by heat, and superfluous and harmful substances have been added as discussed previously in this book. Refined and processed foods are responsible for a large number of health disorders, ranging from headaches to the top 10 leading causes of diseases in this country, and most diets permit these foods to be eaten.

Nothing that man can do to foods, such as high temperature heat treatment, the addition of preservatives, artificial colors and sweeteners, antibiotics (in animal products), and other refined and/or man-made ingredients, can improve the food value of foods over their living food counterparts. To think that it can is ludicrous, since anything done by man to foods (other than necessary harvesting or shipping) alters or adulterates the foods in some way.

The foods that we should eat are not the refined and processed man-made foods that many of us grew up on, including the many fast foods and meat and dairy products that are commonly consumed, but the foods that God made specifically for us to eat, foods that we are biologically suited for, and particularly foods that do not do us harm but good, foods that promote health and longevity.

Grain products, such as bread and cereal, are starchy foods that cause clogging up of the large intestine, or colon. The worst culprits are white flour products such as pastries, pizza dough and while flour bread, but all grain products are starchy, acid-producing foods. The chapters on "The Causes of Arthritis" and "Dangers to Avoid," explain how starchy foods clog up the colon.

The clogging up process contributes to constipation, which is said to be the major precursor of sickness and disease, and, as explained in the chapter on "The Causes of Arthritis," constipation leads to toxicity, which is one of the causes of arthritis. It also hinders the absorption of nutrients in the body, which contributes to nutritional deficiency which is another cause of arthritis.

<u>GMO Crops</u>

Upwards of 75% of the refined and processed foods on supermarket shelves contain GMO products. GMO sweet corn and sugar beets are widely used in refined and processed foods as "sugar" or high-fructose corn syrup (HFCS). GMO soybeans are widely used as soy in many refined and processed foods. Soy is found in almost all baked goods and imitation dairy products, and also in alternative meat products such as veggie burgers. Soy derivatives include hydrolyzed plant protein (HPP), hydrolyzed soy protein (HSP) and/or hydrolyzed vegetable protein (HVP), which are added to a wide range of refined and processed foods, including soda, chips, salad dressings and soups.

GMO (Genetically Modified Organism) refers to a plant or animal (for example, a fish) that is artificially created by inserting genes from one species into the DNA of another species. GE (Genetically Engineered) is another term used for genetically-altered foods.

Many GMO creations have been, and are now being, patented and released into our environment and food supply, and there seems to be no end in sight. Of course, if we buy all our foods "organic", that is, having the proper "Organic" label on them, then we should not have to worry about GMO foods, at least not for the present.

One of the reasons for developing GMO crops was to make them more pesticide- and herbicide-resistant so they could tolerate lethal herbicides and pesticides that non-GMO crops cannot tolerate.

There are two main health concerns associated with consuming GMO crops. First, the highly poisonous pesticides and herbicides that are used on these crops may leave high residues on the crops or seep into the crops themselves. We know that the pesticides and herbicides used on non-GMO crops leave residues and can seep into the crops. See Appendix II.

The second danger is the risk to human health of the Bt (Bacillus thuringiensis) toxin, which is genetically inserted into the DNA of the crop species. The cells of the species that are modified are genetically engineered to include the Bt toxin in order to kill the pests that feed on the crops. The toxin acts as a delayed-action bomb that goes off when pests eat the crops. Crops that have been modified to take the Bt toxin include corn, cotton, and soybeans.

The flurry of reports that were the rage of the 1990s and early 2000s about the health hazards of GMO foods are no longer in the news. The reports have become much less frequent, replaced by carefully-worded reports and articles that are sponsored by food industry advocates of the food industry, that support the continued use of GMO crops.

The principal pro-GMO argument is that GMO crops resist many food viruses and pests, thus making them more available to more people. However, these reports and articles, many of which are on the Web, fail to adequately address, for many people, the earlier-identified dangers of consuming these foods. As a result of these developments, public attention as a whole has shifted away from the dangers of GMOs to other concerns.

There is a scarcity of scientific studies on humans to justify the health risks that are associated with the above-described dangers. But there have been numerous reports showing that human health is adversely affected by these crops. These reports are not limited to the adverse health effects on farm workers who spray the pesticides and herbicides on the crops, but include people who eat the GMO crops.

One of the difficulties in assessing studies done on the human health effects of GMO crops is the fact the evaluation of GE herbicide-resistant crops is conducted by USDA, their evaluation when the crops can be consumed by people is conducted by FDA, while the herbicides are assessed by EPA when there are new potential exposures.[27]

However, it stands to reason that if the strong pesticides and herbicides that are sprayed on GMO crops adversely affect the health of GMO farm workers, then the same poisons may adversely affect the health of people who consume the GMO crops. And, if eating GMO crops that have the Bt toxin kills insects, then eating the crops may adversely affect human health in some way.

At the time of this writing, there are no requirements to label GMO food "GMO" or "GE" or anything else to alert consumers of what they are buying. This is despite opinion polls that show that up to 90 percent of Americans want GMO foods labeled. According to the Center for Food Safety, a national non-profit public interest and environmental advocacy organization, 92% of USA corn, 94% of soybeans and 94% of cotton are genetically engineered.

Foods that are Eaten for Health

Dr. J. C. Jarvis in his book, Arthritis & Folk Medicine, emphasizes the importance of diet when taking cures for diseases, such as arthritis. He calls for eliminating acid-producing foods like those found in ordinary diets, including the vegetarian and vegan diets.

"Biologic food selection is followed every day. This removes wheat foods, wheat cereals, white sugar, citrus fruits and their juices, and muscle meats like beef, lamb, and pork from the daily food intake." - Dr. D. C. Jarvis, *Arthritis & Folk Medicine*.

---

[27] 2016 NCBI report on the Web, entitled, "Human Health Effects of Genetically Engineered Crops."

The Cure for Arthritis

The Creator has blessed and enriched the earth with a wide variety of life-promoting plant foods. It is time we learned about the foods of the plant kingdom and the many tasty and nutritious meals that can be made from them. We have spent too much time and effort learning about the foods of the animal kingdom and how to prepare them, and look what it has cost us in terms of health and lifespan.

We live in a green world. Green is the color of nature, the symbol of youth and growth. Green plants, from lowly grass to lofty trees, together with water, hold the key to life on earth. Even the oceans contain many green plants.

The plant kingdom is a vast reservoir of energy. Plant foods capture the sun's rays and convert their energies into foods for man and beast. Animals cannot convert the energies that are in sun rays directly into energy that can be utilized by the body. The chlorophyll in the leaves of green plants converts sunlight into chemical energy, and we receive this chemical energy when we eat raw plant foods. All animals, including humans, depend on plants to do this for them.

The different wavelengths, or energies, of the sun's electromagnetic energy spectrum are believed to be one of the reasons there are so many different varieties of plants on the earth. It is believed that some plants are more receptive or attuned than others to the different wavelengths. Nutritionists tell us that the more varieties of plant foods we eat, the more we benefit from the different energies.

Each kind of living plant food has its own unique blend of nutrients and life-promoting properties. We can benefit from eating many types of raw plant foods. I believe that the vast variety of plant foods in the world have been given to us for a purpose, and that we can discover that purpose by becoming familiar with these foods.

Just a few examples of the foods that are eaten for health on are given below. Some of these foods are found in ordinary diets, but the mainstays of ordinary diets are meat, dairy and grain products.

Raw fruits and vegetables are eaten regularly on a whole plant food diet, for good reasons. They digest easily and efficiently because their enzymes have not been destroyed by heat. Enzymes have life force properties that Nature intended for us to receive, that support all bodily functions and contain the vitamins and nutrients the body needs for optimum health. Enzymes are further discussed in the chapter on "Dangers to Avoid."

Fruits and vegetables are best eaten when they are ripe. If eaten in their typical store-bought, un-ripened condition, stomachache or some other discomfort is likely. Also, extra energy is required to digest them, and this energy is taken from the energy reserves of the body when it could be used for other purposes, such as healing and self-cleansing.

Fruits and vegetables sold at local food stores are typically shipped-in from distant locations, such as foreign countries, and purposely arrive in an un-ripened condition in order to retard spoilage and prolong shelf-life. To ripen store-bought fruits and vegetables, just set them on the counter tops at home until they are ripe; it usually takes several days, depending on the fruit or vegetable. For example, bananas are typically sold green or partly green in color, unless you happen by the fruit stand right before the bananas are replaced. Ripe bananas are speckled or streaked brown in color, which typically takes several days.

The Cure for Arthritis

Cucumbers are ripe when they are easily flexed. Avocados are ripe when they yield to gentle pressure. Green chilies and jalapenos are ripe when they turn orange or red, do not eat them when they are green. Lemons, limes, oranges and pears are ripe when they are aromatic. Same for red and yellow peppers. Some exceptions to this are apples (all varieties) and root vegetables (for example, carrots, beets, turnips, radishes, potatoes, onions, garlic, etc.). Apples and root vegetables do not ripen to any significant extent after they are picked.

Fruits are nutritious and stimulating, and have many healing qualities. They act to cleanse and energize the cells of the body. I consider fruits to be the ideal food for humankind.

"Fruits alone, even of but one kind, not only heal but nourish perfectly the human body, eliminating entirely the possibility of disease." - Arnold Ehret, *Mucusless Diet Healing System*.

Fatty fruits include avocados and olives. They contain healthy unsaturated fat. Some nutritional experts consider avocado a Superfood, although it is not classified as such. The avocado contains a substantial amount of monounsaturated fats, phytosterols and antioxidants like vitamin E, vitamin C, and carotenoids. It is also high in beta-sitosterol (95 mg per medium-sized avocado) which is known to assist in relieving prostate disorders, such as benign prostatic hyperplasia (BPH).

Plain avocado can be used like butter on raw vegetables such as cabbage, broccoli, cucumber, cauliflower, carrots, asparagus, green onions, tomatoes, chili peppers and celery - with great results. But it's mainly fat, so use avocado in moderation.
The vegetables that have the most tightly compacted layers are some of the most nutritious. They include red and green cabbage, leeks, broccoli, bok choy, green onions, lettuce and celery.

The Cure for Arthritis

Leafy green vegetables, or leafy greens, include spinach, arugula, chard, kale (several varieties), mustard greens, collard greens, turnip greens, parsley, cilantro, lettuce (several varieties), celery greens and dandelion.

Leafy greens are commonly considered vegetables, but I agree with Victoria Boutenko in her book, *Green for Life*, that greens should be their own food group. Greens are the only foods that combine well with all other foods, including other greens. You can't say that about many fruits and vegetables or nuts and seeds.

The chlorophyll in greens strengthens the immune system, helps to detoxify the body and improves digestion. Chlorophyll is rich in antioxidants, minerals, vitamins and readily assimilated enzymes. The chlorophyll in green plants is what converts sunlight into chemical energy, and this energy is made available to us when we eat greens.

Eating a variety of greens ensures that we receive all the amino acids we need in our diets. In his book, *The China Study*, T. Colin Campbell states that plant protein is the healthiest type of protein because it allows for slow but steady synthesis of the proteins.

"Greens are the primary food group that matches human nutritional needs most completely...Chlorophyll is liquefied sun energy. Consuming as much chlorophyll as possible is like bathing our inner organs in sunshine." - Victoria Boutenko, *Green for Life*.

Carrots are high in beta-carotene which is converted to vitamin A in the body. The word "carotene" is derived from the Latin word for carrot, "carota." Nutritional expert Dr. N.W. Walker in his books (see Bibliography), states that raw carrots have all the elements and vitamins that are required by the human body. It could just be that the "lowly carrot" is capable of making up for many of the nutritional deficiencies in the world today.

Carrots are non-starchy vegetables (see the chapter on "Guidelines that Don't Work and Laws that Do.")

Red beets are good for the blood. They lower blood pressure. They improve athletic performance. They are one of the highest of oxygenating foods. Marathon runners are partial to them because they increase their endurance. After consuming red beets, it takes less energy to run a race. This makes red beets important for elderly health, since studies have shown that there is a decline in maximal oxygen consumption with age. In addition, red beets have a high acid-binding rating (see Berg's Tables in Appendix I).

The foods that are best for us are foods that have their life-giving properties intact, that enable the body to withstand the onslaught of diseases, that provide the energy needed for an active and productive life and that promote and sustain optimum health. Nutritional experts agree that a whole plant food diet, such as the raw vegan diet, minimizes bodily toxicity and acidity and rids the body of its toxins better than any other diet.

"Uncooked foods will supply not only all the necessary vitamins and minerals, but also all the enzymes and easily digestible natural starches and proteins needed for healthy functioning of the body." - Paavo O. Airola, N.D., *There is a Cure for Arthritis*.

Healthy eating habits are formed when we accustom the mind to new tastes and food selections found in living plant foods based on reason and knowledge rather than allowing cultural norms and traditions to tell us what foods we should eat or the emotional pulls that certain foods have on us.

The Cure for Arthritis

Detoxification

Detoxification is the process by which the body auto-cleanses itself of toxic wastes. The body is always trying to purge itself of toxins, but certain foods hinder the process. Detoxification really takes off when raw plant foods are consumed exclusively. If you are on an ordinary diet, the detoxification process is, for all practical purposes, ineffectual because ordinary diets cause toxic wastes to build up to the extent where thorough detoxification is not possible. The detoxification process is also known as self-purification or self-cleansing.

Detoxification is the healthy ridding of the body of its accumulated toxins. The process typically causes more frequent defecations and urinations, and maybe some diarrhea. These things are normal and last only during the cleansing process.

Detoxification is how the body heals and rejuvenates itself. Whole plant foods give the body what it needs for self-cleansing and provide it with the best raw materials for cellular reconstruction. Detoxification is the rite of passage everyone must go through to become genuinely healthy. Internal cleansing is required before rejuvenation and optimum health can be achieved.

Toxins accumulate in the organs and tissues of the body from eating animal-based foods, cooked and starchy foods and refined and processed foods. They also accumulate when inorganic multivitamin/mineral supplements are taken, for reasons that have already been discussed. The body also gets toxins from the environment, for example, from exhaust fumes, municipal drinking water, etc.

When the body contains many poisons and is daily given more of them through the foods that are eaten, ill-health reigns. When the body is cleansed of its toxins and is daily given living plant foods, health reigns.

Raw plant foods possess the highest level of nutrients found in any food, and bestow numerous health benefits, some of which are yet to be discussed in this book. An abundance of vitality is available to anyone who adopts the raw vegan diet. When the toxins are removed by the body's self-cleansing process that is enhanced by eating raw plant foods, you feel great.

What is known as "toxic overload" may occur when the detoxification/self-cleansing process is ramped into high gear by a sudden shift, rather than a smooth transition (described later in this chapter), to an all whole plant food diet.

The sudden shift causes an abundance of toxins to be released into the bloodstream all at once, and, as confirmed by many raw food eaters and nutritional experts, this may cause flu or disease like symptoms to occur creating discomfort and malaise. People have gotten seriously ill from transitioning too quickly to a whole plant food diet like the raw vegan diet. This is why a gradual transition to a whole plant food diet is recommended. The purpose of eating some cooked foods during the transition period is to slow down the detoxification process in order to avoid toxic overload.

Living plant foods are so powerful that they immediately start cleansing the body of its poisons. Their life force actions on the body drive out toxic wastes into the bloodstream for their elimination through the normal elimination organs of the body (including the skin). The powers of living plant foods are clearly evidenced by the signs the body gives when it detoxifies itself on these foods.

The Cure for Arthritis

David Wolfe in his book, *The Sunfood Diet Success System*, states that detoxification stops when cooked food is eaten. The dangers associated with cooked foods, why they are detrimental to human health, are described in the chapter on "Dangers to Avoid."

Wastes released into the system from eating a whole plant food diet initially make you feel unhealthy, and during the self-cleansing process you may experience some signs of ill-health. But that is natural and normal. It is caused by the toxins within the tissues and organs of the body being released into the bloodstream. Feelings of fatigue, dizziness, and the signs cited below may be experienced until the "house cleaning" is completed. But when the toxins are eliminated, the feeling of true health is experienced.

The possible ill effects of detoxification should not in any way dissuade the reader from proceeding with a whole plant food diet, since it is the way to true health. They are provided so that you will not be surprised by them when you undergo detoxification.

Normal signs of detoxification include: frequent urinations and/or bowel movements, diarrhea, headaches, runny nose, colds, expectoration, loss of energy, feelings of melancholy, needing more sleep, etc., all indications that the body is purging itself of toxins. Additional signs of detoxification are found in Robert Morse's book, *The Detox Miracle Sourcebook*.

We need to take detoxification into stride when we start eating raw plant foods exclusively. Continue through the healing process trusting that the body is gaining health by what it is doing. Know that drugs that block these symptoms also block the healing process.

The Cure for Arthritis

The transient discomforts of detoxification cause some people to quit a whole plant food diet like the raw vegan diet before the benefits are obtained because they do not understand the detoxification process. But those who stick with the process experience the tremendous boost in vitality that follows self-cleansing, when the accumulated poisons are removed from the system.

"There is only one true healing modality – detoxification. It will bring the body's chemistry back into homeostasis (balance) and remove the toxic metals, elements and substances that don't belong there." - Robert Morse, N.D., *The Detox Miracle Sourcebook*.

Those who have never experienced detoxification cannot know what it is like. You can read about it in books, like this one, and in articles on the Web, but unless you have personally gone through it you will never know what it is like.

"A pure raw plant diet assists the body's cleansing efforts in the most natural way by eliminating any toxicity from entering the system and by simultaneously moving toxicity through the lymph and blood and out the body through the eliminating organs (the bowels, kidneys, liver, skin, sinuses and lungs). A purification of the diet enforces a self-healing and radical whole-body rejuvenation." - David Wolfe, *The Sunfood Diet Success System*.

In my opinion, the chief importance of detoxification is to relieve the body of its burden of constipation, to remove the coating of paste-like plaque that has formed on the walls of the intestines after years of eating the wrong foods, foods detrimental to health (see the chapter on "Dangers to Avoid.")

One of the things I learned during my first year on the raw vegan diet that was not covered in the books listed in the Bibliography, was that improper, or bad, food combinations can cause not only stomachache, headache, heartburn, and flatulence, but also constipation.

Antioxidants

Antioxidants are substances that protect the cells of the body against the effects of free radicals. Antioxidants neutralize free radicals. Antioxidants include beta-carotene, lycopene, p-coumaric acid, and vitamins A, C, and E (alpha-tocopherol), all of which are found in raw plant foods.

A free radical is a molecule that with an unpaired electron. It is "free" to react "radically" with other molecules and cause cellular disruption and damage.

According to the National Cancer Institute, damage to the cells of the body caused by free radicals play an important role in the development of cancer and other serious health disorders.

Antioxidants are the body's main defenses against free radicals. They neutralize free radicals by chemically combining them with the molecules in the foods. As discussed in the chapter on "The Causes of Arthritis," foods that are rich in antioxidants are known to stop or reverse toxic buildup.

We should eat foods that are high in antioxidants. The foods of the raw vegan diet are rich in enzymes, nutrients and antioxidants. Whole plant foods that are particularly rich in antioxidants are listed below.

WHOLE PLANT FOODS HIGH IN ANTIOXIDANTS

Fruits – all kinds

The Cure for Arthritis

Green leafy vegetables (Greens) -- all kinds
Vegetables – all kinds
Spices and herbs
Superfoods

It is important to eat as many antioxidant-rich foods as we can to strengthen the immune system, neutralize the poisons within the body and stop or reverse toxic buildup in the body.

Most antioxidants are destroyed by heat. While freezing seems to preserve antioxidant activity, heating adversely affects almost all antioxidants. This means, for example, that canned and jarred fruits and vegetables, which have been heat treated during refining and processing, have significantly lower levels of antioxidants than their living food counterparts. It indicates that fruits and vegetables that are fast-frozen are acceptable to eat on the raw vegan diet.

A whole plant food diet is the best assurance anyone can have of getting the antioxidants that are needed for health.

Oxidative stress occurs when an imbalance exists between free radical activity and antioxidant activity in the body. An ordinary diet, such as the Standard American Diet, causes oxidative stress which contributes to aging and degenerative diseases. It is known that when foods contain insufficient antioxidants to counteract free radicals, the resulting imbalance can damage the DNA and the proteins and fatty tissues of the body.

Researchers have shown that mental stress creates free radicals. Radiation, environmental pollutants, such as smog, cigarette smoke, car exhaust fumes and impurities and toxins in municipal drinking water, also create free radicals.

Agricultural chemicals are known to destroy the antioxidants in crops. Therefore, it is wise to eat organic produce to maximize the antioxidants we receive from natural plant foods.

According to Dr. Michael Greger's book, *How Not To Die*, antioxidant supplements, such as vitamin C and beta carotene, do not work. The body needs to get its antioxidants from living plant foods.

The ORAC (Oxygen Radical Absorbance Capacity) is considered a useful antioxidant rating system, although it is not the only one.

ORAC was used by the USDA until 2012, which, according to the Web, was the year USDA's Nutrient Data Laboratory (NDL) removed the ORAC Database for Selected Foods from the NDL website. It was removed due to pressure on the USDA from independent laboratories that argued that "in vitro" tests do not conclusively reflect what happens in the human body. It is uncertain whether the pressure was due to legitimate concerns or based on the biased opinion of the meat and dairy industries. However, it appears to be a somewhat specious argument since measuring the effect of antioxidants in the human body is not possible, according to papers published on the Web at the time of this writing.

Nevertheless, ORAC is still used by many nutritionists as a comparative basis for antioxidant capacity since it reflects how effectively a food or product neutralizes free radicals as measured by the degradation of a fluorescent dye. ORAC is a particularly useful measure of the antioxidant effectiveness of foods that contain complex ingredients with both slow- and fast-acting antioxidants, and also foods that have combined or synergistic effects.

ORAC ratings of various herbs and spices, taken from the Web at the time of this writing, are listed below.

SAMPLE OF ORAC ANTIOXIDANT RATINGS

Cloves, ground	314, 446
Cinnamon, ground	267, 536
Oregano, dried	200,129
Rosemary, dried	165, 280
Parsley, dried	73, 670

Many foods that are commonly eaten today, such as meat- and dairy-based foods, have, in comparison to the above values, negligible ORAC ratings, which indicates low antioxidant effectiveness. These foods include, but are not limited to, salmon with an ORAC rating of 30, eggs (20), hot dogs (300), McDonald's Crispy Chicken Sandwich (180), Little Caesar's Cheese Pizza (180), and fried chicken (50).

At the time of this writing, a complete listing of ORAC ratings of many foods is available on the following website:

https://www.superfoodly.com/orac-values/

It should be noted that the ORAC rating is based on 100 grams of food. Since raw fruits and vegetables, including fresh (undried) herbs, have water content, the ORAC ratings of these foods are much lower than their dried alternatives. If this is not considered, the ORAC ratings of raw fruits and vegetables can be misleading.

When we eat living plant foods, the body is provided with all the nutrients it needs for optimum health, including Nature's own antioxidants. The body's defenses against free radicals are the greatest when we eat raw plant foods, which means the immune system is strengthened by these foods.

Antioxidant supplements, such as the vitamin C and beta carotene supplements that are available today, are not good sources for the antioxidants the body needs. A whole plant food diet is the best assurance that anyone can have of getting the antioxidants needed for health.

The Immune System

The body's ability to fight illnesses is determined by the health of the immune system. Certain diseases, including cancer, suppress the immune system and allow increased attacks by unfriendly microbes, which, as stated previously, include the smallest of microbes, the viruses. Nutritionists tell us that the best way to improve the health of the immune system is to eat plenty of whole plant foods.

Raw plant foods have a benign and beneficial effect on the entire organism. After eating raw plant foods exclusively for only a short time, the body ramps up its self-cleansing process and focuses more on healing. Raw plant foods enhance the health of the immune system. Raw foodists throughout the world have been cleansed and healed of their health disorders, and remain in health, by the powers of raw plant foods. These powers are made available to anyone who adopts a whole plant food diet, such as the raw vegan diet.

True health, which is health in tune with Nature, is gained when we adopt a whole plant food diet and reduce the quantity of the foods eaten. It is then that the body's self-healing process is fully engaged to produce true health. It is then, too, that the health of the immune system is greatest. When true health arrives, it is like a sunrise after a long night, the kind of health you may never have experienced before.

As discussed above, antioxidants are substances that protect the cells of the body against the effects of free radicals, and they are found in abundance in raw plant foods.

<u>Transitioning to a Whole Plant Food Diet</u>

If you have been on an ordinary diet, such as the Standard American Diet, for a long time, as most people have, it may be best to gradually transition to a whole plant food diet, although the shift in diets can occur much quicker. There are reasons for this as were explained in the above section on "Detoxification."

Eliminating all meat and dairy products, refined sugar and refined salt from your diet is a huge step in the right direction. It will be your first goal if you are not already there. It means stop eating fast foods, including energy drinks, sodas and colas, most restaurant foods and refined and processed foods.

In the place of meat and dairy products, eat raw fruits, vegetables and leafy greens, and get used to them. Then expand your food selections to include different varieties than those you are already used to. Start using natural, unrefined sea salt (see the chapter on "Salt.")

Anyone can improve their health today simply by quitting one or two harmful foods or ingredients and replacing them with healthier choices. Then, after several weeks, declare victory and move on to quit another food or ingredient, replacing it with a healthier choice. In this way, you progress to the whole plant food diet.

Get to where you are eating at least one meal a day of only raw fruit and maybe also greens (for example, a green smoothie for breakfast). Raw fruits counteract many of the harmful effects of a mixed diet, that is, a cooked food and raw food diet. Eating more raw fruit (fresh or sun-dried) will be of benefit to the cells of the body and will enhance the self-cleansing process.

It is during the transition period that the food combination laws, which are described in the chapter on "Guidelines that Don't Work and Laws that Do," are learned. Plan on making mistakes; it's part of any learning experience. For a more complete discussion about the many things that are learned when transitioning to a whole plant food diet, and for how to clear the final hurdle, which is quitting cooked foods, see the book, *The Powers that Heal*, which is listed in the Bibliography.

Additional Benefits of Eating Whole Plant Foods

Raw plant foods lower body mass index (BMI), meaning body fat, which results in decreased risks of high blood pressure, elevated serum cholesterol, cardiovascular disease, type 2 diabetes and cancers. A plant-based diet is the only diet that has been shown to reverse diseases. Examples are ischemic heart disease (i.e., insufficient blood supply) and type 2 diabetes. The research conducted by Dr. Caldwell Esselstyn, Jr. on how raw plant foods prevent and reverse heart disease Is well known and was described previously in this chapter.

"The foods you consume can heal you faster and more profoundly than the most expensive prescription drugs, and more dramatically than the most extreme surgical interventions, with only positive side effects. They can prevent cancer, heart disease, Type 2 diabetes, stroke, macular degeneration, migraines, erectile dysfunction, and arthritis – and that's only the short list." - T. Colin Campbell and Howard Jacobson, *Whole, Rethinking the Science of Nutrition*.

As previously discussed in the chapter on "The Causes of Arthritis," acidity is a blood condition mainly brought on by eating acid-forming foods, such as bread, meat and dairy products, fatty foods, refined and processed foods (canned, jarred, etc.), fast foods and restaurant foods. According to leading nutritionists, acid-forming foods are responsible for many of the health issues and diseases that are prevalent in the world today, including arthritis, diabetes and kidney failure.

The body is the greatest healing machine. It only requires the right foods to accomplish what it alone knows how to do. When living plant foods are eaten in place of dead, cooked foods, the body receives the amazing ionic and magnetic properties of living foods as well as their potent, unaltered natural minerals, vitamins and enzymes.

Healthy people, healthy animals and healthy plants do not get sick. But health is not to be had for the asking. If it were, everyone would be extraordinarily healthy. Rather, it must be earned. Food habits must be changed for the body to rid itself of the causes of ill-health, including arthritis.

The beacon of warning, the clarion call for proper action, has been sent out. We need to become more our own doctors than ever before, and the sooner it starts the better it will be for us, not only as individuals, but as a society, to avoid the unnecessary suffering associated with medical treatments that are not designed to heal our maladies or prevent them from recurring, but instead are prescribed for relieving their symptoms.

The Cure for Arthritis

Much of what has been discussed up to this point has provided clues about what should be done to cure arthritis. One of the things that must be done is to reduce or eliminate the intake of certain foods and food products from our diets, and replace them with healthier choices. But other things should also be done, as discussed in this chapter.

The cure for arthritis is a combination of practices that attack the underlying causes of the disease, reverse the damage done by the disease, and prevent the disease from spreading to other parts of the body. Many of the practices have already been discussed. Each, by itself, is known to reduce the pains and inflammation of arthritis. Combined, they work to ensure an effective and permanent cure.

1. Reduce or eliminate from the diet foods that cause acidity and toxicity in the body, such as meat and dairy products and refined and processed foods, including fast foods and drinks. In their place, eat whole plant foods, such as raw fruits and vegetables, and drink water. These changes alone result in remarkable improvements in arthritic conditions.

Stopping the intake of acid-causing foods, and eating foods that are nutrient rich and low in acid, addresses two of the underlying causes of arthritis, nutrient deficiency and bodily acidity.

The more we eat whole plant foods, the more effective is the cure.

"To the degree that foods are used in their completely natural state, without treatment or processing, are they adapted to support life and maintain immunity to disease." - Arnold Paul De Vries.

Moving towards a whole plant food diet day by day helps all suffers of arthritis to reduce their symptoms, no matter what type of arthritis they may have. This is confirmed not only by the many nutritionists and nutrition-minded medical doctors who support this treatment, many of which are referenced in this book, but by the personal experiences of many arthritics.

2. Avoid mineral supplementation. Instead, get your minerals from whole plant foods. Many websites can assist in this process.

Most of the mineral supplements on the market are made of compounds of inorganic minerals, including calcium carbonate, calcium boron gluconate, magnesium oxide, zinc carbonate and zinc gluconate. As explained in this book, inorganic minerals are not properly utilized by the body, if utilized at all, and that the body treats these minerals as toxins, and what cannot be purged from the system ends up in the joints and tissues of the body.

Calcium, boron, magnesium, zinc and many other minerals needed by the body are found in living plant foods in organic form. Examples of these foods are leafy green vegetables, including collard greens, turnip greens, chard, kale and cabbage, root vegetables, such as carrots, turnips, onions, radishes and potatoes; seeds and nuts; grains and legumes; and sea vegetables, such as kelp and dulse. On a whole plant food diet, the body gets all the minerals it needs. If it is still believed that more calcium is needed, then ensure that the calcium supplements taken are derived from plant foods, because plants convert minerals taken up from the soil and water into organic form.

3. Reduce or eliminate the consumption of refined salts. Refined salts, including table salt and refined sea salt, are heat-treated to very high temperatures during their refining and processing which alters the chemical structure of the salts and makes them unsuitable for the body. This is described in more detail in the chapter on "Salt."

Refined salts are found in almost all refined and processed foods. They are added to many packaged natural fruit and vegetable foods that are sold in supermarkets, such as freshly diced or minced fruits and vegetables. Checking ingredients and watching your salt intake at home greatly reduces the daily intake of refined salts. Refined salt is typically listed in the ingredients as "Salt" or "Sea Salt."

As stated in the chapter on "The Importance of Alternative Medicine," Dr. Ann Wigmore healed herself of arthritis by going on a whole plant food diet and eliminating table salt from her diet.

Natural sea salt, such as Celtic Sea Salt, which is a North Atlantic Ocean sun-evaporated salt, has not undergone heat treatment other than being heated by the sun to evaporate the water. It has no additives or preservatives, and is not blanched white like refined salts, but has a natural greyish or pinkish cast to it. It may be an acceptable alternative to refined salt, as explained in the chapter on "Salt."

4. Drink diluted apple cider vinegar (ACV) sweetened with honey twice daily in the recommended proportions. As discussed in the chapter on "The Importance of Alternative Medicine," ACV assists the body in removing the hard acid and mineral deposits from the joints. The recommended proportions, and the types of ACV and honey to use were provided in that chapter.

The Cure for Arthritis

It is noted, as explained in the chapter on "My Story," that higher than recommended concentrations of ACV can cause an acidic blood condition, which is one of the things the cure is preventing. In addition, higher than recommended concentrations of ACV can irritate the esophagus and/or damage tooth enamel.

5. If possible, drink distilled water rather than faucet or bottled water, and use it in the ACV drink. Distilled water does not contain minerals, and, as explained in this book, it helps to dissolve the hard acid and mineral deposits from the joints and tissues of the body so that they can be released into the bloodstream for elimination.

It is noted that, as explained in the chapter on "Distilled Water" and elsewhere in the book, distilled water does not leach out needed minerals from the body, but only helps remove unneeded minerals.

Parts 4 and 5 above help to reverse the damage already done by the disease and prevent the disease from spreading to other parts of the body.

6. Exercise the affected joints daily to help break up the hard acid and mineral deposits, including calcium crystals, that have formed in the joints. Exercising the joints works to improve joint range of motion, helps to strengthen the supporting muscles and keep the ligaments and tendons flexible. It may also increase the production of synovial fluid, which can improve joint function.

Exercising of the joints should not be overdone, but some type of bending or twisting is recommended. Painful at first, it gets less painful as time goes by on the cure. Examples of proper exercises to use may be seen on Yoga websites, for example, yoga exercises for the hands and feet.

7. Positive thinking enhances the cure. It is important to believe in what one is doing. That is why a knowledge of the causes of arthritis and the importance of foods and nutrition in bodily healing should precede dietary change and the implementation of the cure. Have faith in the cure, in yourself, and in Nature, and things will turn around in a relatively short time.

It is what you are capable of doing now that counts. Put your trust in the efficacy of the cure, and the powers that heal will deliver the victory to you soon.

When the cure has been implemented, the body soon adjusts itself to the changes and starts the long-awaited healing and recovery process. The time it takes for healing to occur depends on the extent of damage that has been done by the disease, including bone deformities, which correlates with the kind of diet that has been practiced, and how long it has been practiced prior to beginning the cure. It also depends on how long a healthy diet has been practiced, one that does not support the underlying causes of the disease.

Although some people see improvement in their condition in a relatively short time, one should not expect to reverse the results of a lifetime of improper eating habits overnight, or in a matter of days or weeks. However, pain relief comes in a much shorter time than it took for the pains and inflammation of arthritis to develop.

In my case, for example, I had eaten an ordinary diet for a large part of my life, and had suffered from the pains and inflammation of osteoarthritis for over seven years, before taking the cure. But when the cure was fully implemented, it took only weeks to see improvement in my condition, several months to see the pains and inflammation subside considerably, and a little longer for them to become negligible to where they were no longer affecting my lifestyle.

As you continue with the cure, seeing positive results will encourage you to stick with it until it has performed its work.

In his book, *Arthritis & Folk Medicine*, Dr. D. C. Jarvis states that the diluted ACV drink can, by itself, cure arthritis, but seldom in a period of less than three months, and sometimes it takes more than eighteen months. He also states that some people who have taken the ACV and honey treatment have experienced improvements in their arthritic condition within a matter of days. While this may not be the case with most people, and it was not true in my case, it shows what this part of the treatment can do.

As related in Margaret Hills' book, *Treating Arthritis: The Drug-Free Way*, after six weeks of her treatment, which consisted of eating a nutritious, low-acid diet and drinking diluted ACV, the majority of her patients reported considerably less pain and a general feeling of well-being that they had not experienced in years.

Nature is not on the 9:15 PM express to the suburbs. She does not rush, but takes her time as necessary to complete her work. The damage done to the system from years of unintentional wrong eating requires correction by the body's self-cleansing process before improvements are noticeable.

As explained in the chapter on "How to Change the Situation," transitioning from an ordinary diet to a healthy whole plant food diet involves many things, such as giving up certain foods and eating healthier foods. Important steps along the way include eliminating meat and dairy products, sugary drinks, refined and processed foods and refined salt, and substituting in their place raw fruits and vegetables, nuts and seeds and natural, unrefined sea salt.

The body always lets us know how we are treating it. Whenever food choices or food combinations cause discomfort, such as stomachache or headache, we should do something about it to prevent it from happening again. The laws of proper food combining apply to any kind of diet. The laws are discussed in the chapter on "Guidelines that Don't Work and Laws that Do." Additional information is provided in the chapter on "My Story."

While on the cure, there may be occasional flareups of the pains. Adjust the diet accordingly, because the foods or food products being consumed, including mustard and ketchup which are loaded with unrefined salt, are very probably responsible, causing excess acidity and/or toxicity.

The cure eliminates, or greatly reduces, the pains and inflammation of acute and chronic arthritis without exacting payment in the form of drawbacks or downsides. It also prevents the symptoms from returning and spreading to other parts of the body. While occasional flareups of pains may occur during the cure, they are, as discussed, feedback signals the body gives that indicate a need to change something about the foods or food products that are being consumed.

Drugs are not necessary on the cure, and may hinder its success. Nutritionists tell us that drugs that block the symptoms of arthritis also block the healing process. If the natural self-healing process is repressed through medication (drugs), and we continue the consumption of foods and drinks that are harmful to the body, then the cure is thwarted. Healing does not come from drugs. It comes from natural bodily processes, such as self-cleansing or detoxification that remove accumulated toxins, obstructions and acidosis from the body, from rest, and from providing the body with the nourishment it needs.

"Remember, it took years to build-up your arthritis condition, so don't expect overnight clean-up miracles. Work with Mother Nature and be patient as she is with you." - Paul C. and Patricia Bragg, *Water, The Shocking Truth That Can Save Your Life*.

Surprisingly, however, at the time of this writing, the cure was virtually unrecognized by the popular media, including the Internet, television, newspapers, magazines, and many books about arthritis. To be perfectly fair about it because some reports may have been missed in the review of popular media sources, I should say that the cure, at the time of this writing, has been underreported by the media. Also, to the best of my knowledge, the cure has not received governmental support, and is not being used by the mainstream medical profession. After taking the cure, you may wonder why all this is so.

The chapters that follow provide information that will assist the reader in curing their arthritis.

Dangers to Avoid

This chapter is not intended to discuss dangers caused or imposed by the loss of mobility or strength that accompanies arthritis, but rather dangers that should be avoided that worsen the condition. Each is known to worsen an arthritic condition since each contributes to the underlying causes of arthritis.

Saturated Fats

Saturated fats are fats that are solid at room temperature. These fats are found in all animal products, including meat, dairy, fish and poultry products, and also in many refined and processed foods, such as canned foods that contain animal fat and/or palm oil. Saturated fats are not found to any great extent in plant foods, but there are two exceptions, palm oil and coconut.

Saturated fats in animal products are typically long-chain fatty acids that are difficult to breakdown, or assimilate, in the body. The amount of saturated fat found in most animal products is typically about 30-50%. Palm oil is about 50% saturated fat.

Medical experts agree that saturated fats raise the levels of LDL (bad) cholesterol, which increases the risk of cardiovascular disease.

A 2017 study published in the Wiley Online Library[28] reported that saturated fats change the composition of cartilage, particularly the

---

[28] A Queensland University of Technology study entitled, "Dietary Fats and Osteoarthritis: Insights, Evidences and New Horizons," by Sunderajhan Sekar, Yin Xiao, et al.

cartilage in the joints. The results of the study implicate common dietary fatty acids, such as those found in meat and dairy products, with the development and worsening of arthritic conditions. The study involved following more than 2,000 patients with OA for up to four years. It found that those who ate the most fatty foods showed increased joint cartilage damage compared with those who ate healthy fats, such as those found in avocados and olives.

Professor Xiao, one of authors of the report, stated that the findings suggest that it's not wear and tear, but diet, that has a lot to do with the onset of osteoarthritis.

To get the saturated fats we need on the whole plant food diet, olives, coconut, avocado, and nuts and seeds may be eaten. These foods are low in saturated fats. Nuts come from trees[29]. The saturated fat in coconuts is a medium-chain fatty acid, which, unlike the long-chain fatty acids found in animal products, is easily assimilated by the body[30]. Also, coconut does not elevate LDL blood cholesterol levels.

Whole plant foods that contain saturated fat have many healthy benefits, such as protecting the body against heart disease and stroke, and certain whole plants foods, such as coconut, have the ability to neutralize or eradicate Candida and other pathogenic microorganisms.

Professor Sunder Sekar, one of the authors of the above

---

[29] The peanut, which is not really a nut, but a legume, grows in the ground.

[30] Coconut oil, the kind typically sold in bottles, is a fractionated oil that is known to raise cholesterol levels in people, per Victoria Boutenko's book, Raw & Beyond. Fractionated oils also include other so-called "healthy" oils, such as olive oil and avocado oil. It is best to stay away from fractionated oils.

referenced report, tested lauric acid, a saturated fatty acid found in coconut oil. He stated in the report, "Interestingly, when we replaced the meat fat in the diet with lauric acid, we found decreased signs of cartilage deterioration and metabolic syndrome, so it seems to have a protective effect."

A conclusion of the report was that it is not wear and tear, but diet, that has a lot to do with the onset of osteoarthritis.

It is noted that the American Heart Association recommends a daily saturated fat intake of no more than 5-6% calories, or about 13 grams, which is a very small amount of saturated fat. Their recommendation essentially means cutting out all animal-based foods and eating very little, if any, whole plant foods that contain saturated fat.

Cooked Foods

Nutritional experts have stressed for years that cooked foods are harmful to human health, and that the cooking of foods done at home and in restaurants, and in the food factories that manufacture canned, bottled and jarred foods, reduces the food value of the foods by altering their chemical properties and destroying important food constituents such as enzymes and nutrients, which also includes vitamins. They have also been telling us that cooked foods of almost any kind create acidity in the body.

Cooked foods create acidity in the body, whereas uncooked (raw) plant foods alkalize the body. As explained in the chapter on "The Causes of Arthritis," acidity is a major cause of arthritis. Cooked foods also cause constipation, which, as also explained in the chapter on "The Causes of Arthritis," leads to toxicity, another cause of arthritis. In addition, constipation hinders the absorption of nutrients in the body, which contributes to nutritional deficiency, yet another cause of arthritis.

It is now known that cooking and the refining and processing of foods are responsible for the development of many of the sicknesses and diseases that plague humankind.

As stated previously, Americans eat more cooked food than any people on earth, and spend more money on doctor bills and healthcare than any people on earth. The fast food franchises, as well as other eating establishments, grill, fry, bake, and steam-heat their foods, or use dehydrated foods that have already been refined and processed using these methods.

Robert Morse in his book, *The Detox Miracle Sourcebook*, explains how cooking dramatically decreases the molecular energy of foods, since heat affects the electrons of the food molecules and alters their molecular structure. However, when we eat raw plant foods, their high electromagnetic energy is transferred to the body and its cells.

Dr. N. W. Walker in many of his books, such as *Colon Health* and *Become Younger*, tells us that foods are demagnetized when they are cooked, and that only living (raw, uncooked) plant foods have the magnetic properties that are needed by the body. He states that the fiber we consume in our diets should be comprised of the fiber or roughage of raw plant foods, and that if this fiber comes from cooked foods, it will be demagnetized, or devitalized, to the extent that it will pass through the system with little or no benefit.

In addition, cooked, starchy foods leave a plaster-like coating on the walls of the large intestine (colon). This coating builds up over time as more of these foods are consumed, which decreases the capacity to absorb vital nutrients and prevents food from being completely digested. More is provided about this in the next section of this chapter.

Cooked food is any food heated above 118° F. It includes almost every kind of food that comes in an airtight sealed package (bag, box, can, jar, bottle, etc.). For comparison purposes, a hot shower is 105° F, typical pasteurization temperature is 160° F, water boils at 212° F, canned foods are heated during the canning process to 240-250° F, and microwave and stove ovens heat foods to 300-500° F.

"Cooked food is dead, and actually unsuitable as nourishment for the digestive processes of all animals, including human beings." - Dr. Ann Wigmore, *Be Your Own Doctor.*

Cooked foods (plant or animal) are foods devoid of life. They require additional energy from the body to be digested and assimilated, energy that could be used for other purposes, such as healing. Cooked foods contain coagulated and unusable proteins and dead enzymes that are toxic to the body.

According to Dr. D. C. Jarvis in his book, *Folk Medicine*, cooking reduces potassium 70% for carrots, onions, potatoes, pumpkin and spinach, 60% for cauliflower, cabbage, peas, asparagus, string beans and Brussel sprouts, and 50% for corn, beets and tomatoes. Potassium is needed for the proper functioning of the nervous system.

Cooked foods are tasteless compared to raw foods, which is why they require condiments, such as salt, pepper and sugar, and combinations of them. Many of the condiments have deleterious effects on the body, including refined sugar and refined salt, as explained in this book.

The Cure for Arthritis

Because cooked foods are dead foods and deficient in nutrients, our hunger is not sated when we eat them in small portions, so we overeat. However, overeating is known to be a precursor of many health complications, including obesity and disease.

As stated previously, raw plant foods are foods as-found in nature. They are not cooked or chemically altered, and they do not contain preservatives, artificial colors or flavors. Raw plant foods are living foods with their natural life force properties intact. It is this life force that is imparted to us when we eat raw plant foods.

The dangers of cooked foods discussed so far are sufficient in themselves to justify eliminating all cooked foods from your diet. But cooking of foods has more dangers.

As discussed in the chapter on "How to Change the Situation," if food is browned by heat treatment, such as by broiling, baking or deep frying, dangerous chemicals are created, such as advanced glycation end-products (AGEs), which have been linked to diabetes and heart disease.

Furthermore, nutritional experts assert that cooked food is addictive. Like other addictions, the cooked food addiction gets stronger with continued use.

The consensus of modern nutritional experts, including Norman W. Walker, Robert Morse, Arnold Ehret, Theresa Mitchell, Ann Wigmore, Edward Howell, David Wolfe, Herbert M. Shelton, O.L.M. Abramowski, Fred Hirsch, Harvey Diamond, Bernard Jensen, Professor Spira, Kristina Carrillo-Bucaram, Victoria Boutenko, Joe Alexander and Paavo Airola, is that the consumption of cooked foods is detrimental to human health, and that they should not be eaten.

Because enzymes are a principal food component that is destroyed when food is cooked, they merit additional discussion.

The Vital Importance of Enzymes

Enzymes are life-force factors, biological catalysts that are necessary for life processes. They are substances that make life possible. Enzymes are needed for every chemical reaction that takes place in the body. It is claimed that no mineral, vitamin or hormone can do any work without enzymes. The body's ability to digest and assimilate foods is totally dependent on enzymes.

"I attest that the kitchen stove and its big brothers, the heat treatment machinery in food factories, are responsible for destroying a whole category of food elements, namely the heat-sensitive exogenous food enzymes." - Dr. Edward Howell, *Enzyme Nutrition.*

Raw plant foods are replete with enzymes as provided by nature to facilitate their digestion and assimilation in the body. According to Dr. Edward Howell, raw plant foods have all the enzymes needed for human consumption. The pancreas produces enzymes, but you'll always have exogenous enzymes if you eat raw, uncooked foods.

"To get enzymes from food, one must eat raw food. The heat used in cooking destroys all food enzymes and forces the organism to produce more enzymes, thus enlarging digestive organs, especially the pancreas." - Dr. Edward Howell, *Enzyme Nutrition.*

The nutritional experts believe that eating cooked food requires the body to use up its enzyme reserves for digestion and assimilation. More specifically, the enzymes of the body must perform the job of digesting cooked foods. This depletes the enzyme reserves of the body, making it increasingly difficult as time goes by to properly digest foods. As a result, we become weaker and more fatigued, despite the amount of food we consume. In addition, energy that is used by the body to digest cooked foods is diverted away from other badly needed bodily functions such as self-cleansing and healing.

One of the things that interests me in particular about the dangers of eating cooked foods is that Dr. Howell in his book, *Enzyme Nutrition,* states that enzyme activity in the body becomes weaker with age. He also states that based on clinical studies performed on animals and humans, each of us is given a limited supply of enzymes at birth, and that when the supply is depleted, we die, and the faster we use up our enzyme supply the shorter our life will be. This is one of the main reasons why we should avoid all cooked foods. It implies that the more cooked foods we eat, the sooner our life will come to an end.

Again, cooked foods are devoid of enzymes because heat destroys them. Furthermore, cooked foods cause us to look older than we really are. They make wrinkles appear, especially on the face. Want to look young? Eat raw plant foods. Want to look old? Eat cooked foods.

Dr. Ann Wigmore, in her book, *Be Your Own Doctor,* states that when food is cooked it permits tumors and cancer growth to build, but when food is eaten raw the cancer and other growths immediately begin to shrink. This indicates that cooked foods are precursors of human disease.

Surprisingly, there is a dearth of information on the Web about the harmful effects of cooked foods on human health. Many of the websites queried for this information actually *encourage* eating cooked and starchy foods as part of a healthy diet. Again, books have the answers to many of the important questions about foods and nutrition.

Raw plant foods may be sliced, diced, run through a food processor, blender, etc., as long as they are not cooked. They can be eaten by themselves or combined with other raw foods if properly combined (see chapter on "Guidelines that Don't Work and Laws that Do").

"Eating raw foods is the number one activity which preserves enzymes and maximizes health." - Gabriel Cousens, *Conscious Eating*.

The conclusion is obvious. We should eat as many enzyme-rich foods as possible, which are raw plant foods, and avoid all cooked foods.

Vegetables that are so often cooked can be eaten raw. We can eat raw potatoes, as long as we don't eat green ones that can be toxic. Also, there are plenty of raw plant foods that satisfy cravings for cooked foods and sweets. For example, what is more satisfying than a ripe peach or mango? You can snack on pecans and honey, cacao nibs or bee pollen soaked in water, bananas with Mission figs or dates and sweet apples.

Substituting living plant foods for cooked foods solves all of the problems described in this chapter.

For more information about how cooked foods are harmful to human health, I refer you to the books listed in the Bibliography by Norman W. Walker, Robert Morse, Arnold Ehret, Theresa Mitchell, Ann Wigmore, Edward Howell, David Wolfe, Herbert M. Shelton, O.L.M. Abramowski, Fred Hirsch, Harvey Diamond, Bernard

The Cure for Arthritis

Jensen, Professor Spira, Kristina Carrillo-Bucaram, Victoria Boutenko, Joe Alexander and Paavo Airola.

The dangers of eating cooked foods may shock or surprise many people because most of us grew up eating cooked foods and have learned to like them. Hopefully, this chapter will serve as a re-thinking starting point about how cooked foods should be viewed.

"If you eat living food, the same will quicken you, but if you kill your food the dead food will kill you also. For life comes only from life, and from death always comes death." - Attributed to Jesus, *The Essene Gospel of Peace, Book One*.

Starchy Foods

Many of the contributors to our understanding of the causes of human diseases were famous nutritionists, including Professor Arnold Ehret, who was popular in Germany in the early 1900s, and later in America.

Ehret was probably the first scientist to recognize that mucus-forming foods cause waste obstruction in the body, and that the obstruction causes disease. In his book, *The Cause and Cure of Human Illness*, he states that there are two main reasons for human disease: 1) constipation caused by mucus-producing foods, and 2) overeating, that is, eating more than is necessary, more than the system can handle, more than it actually needs.

As explained in the chapter on "The Causes of Arthritis," starchy foods create acidity in the body. Acidity is a major cause of arthritis. Starchy foods also cause a plaster-like coating to form on the inner walls of the large intestine, or colon, that builds up to where it restricts, or even obstructs, the passage of wastes out of the system. The constipation leads to toxicity, another cause of arthritis. In addition, constipation hinders the absorption of nutrients in the body, which contributes to nutritional deficiency, yet another cause of arthritis.

In his landmark book, *The Mucusless Diet Healing System*, first published in 1922, Ehret released to the world his incredible findings about how optimum health can be achieved by eating a starch-free diet consisting of fresh raw fruits, leafy greens and non-starchy vegetables (mucusless foods) which he claimed was the optimal diet for human health. The book is considered by many nutritional experts to be the definitive work on the prevention and curing of human disease through diet and fasting.

Starchy foods include wheat, corn, rice, white and red potatoes, beans of all kinds and peas. They also include food products made from these foods, such as bread, pasta, cereals, pastries, corn starch, etc. (Note that carrots and beets are non-starchy foods as discussed in the chapter on "Guidelines that Don't Work and Laws that Do").

Many nutritional experts agree that starchy foods cause disease in the human body because of the constipation resulting from the paste-like plaque that forms, or plates-out, on the insides of the large intestine, or colon. They believe that people are nutrient deficient and constipated because of the large amounts of starchy foods they habitually consume.

The clogging up process resulting from the consumption of starchy foods can be easily proven on the raw vegan diet by simply eating white flour products, such as pizza or while flour bread, for several days. The result is constipation and difficult bowel movements, whereas stopping the consumption of these foods results in the return of regular and smooth defecations.

The Cure for Arthritis

The clogging up of the intestines caused by starchy foods causes intestinal bacteria to multiply inordinately which releases poisons into the blood stream. The state of constipation is the primary cause of illness and disease in the human body, according to Dr. N. W. Walker, Arnold Ehret, Dr. Ann Wigmore, Fred Hirsch, Karyn Calabrese, Professor Spira, and other nutritionists.

The degree of being constipated correlates with the number of meals eaten per day versus the number of defecations per day. In other words, if a person is not having as many bowel movements per day as meals taken per day, they are constipated, and the lower the ratio the more constipated they are.

Dr. N. W. Walker found that the plaster-like coating formed by starchy foods builds up and increases in thickness over time until only a small opening remains in the large intestine for food residue to pass out of the system. This conclusion is based on Walker's examination of thousands of X-rays of the colons of chronically ill patients. He believed that starchy foods were primarily responsible for this obstruction of the colon and the resulting spread of poisons throughout the body.

Walker believed that any treatment of disease would be totally ineffective unless the accumulated starchy plaque that has formed in the large intestine over the years has been washed out of the colon by colonic irrigations. This conclusion is based on his healing of chronically ill patients by having them undergo a series of colonics. It was the cleansing action of the colonics that caused the plaque to be released from the walls of the colon, and when that occurred the health of his patients was restored. This is exactly what Arnold Ehret and others have stressed in their books.

Most people are not aware of the dangers of starchy foods, as they are not aware of the dangers of cooked foods. At the time of this writing, I could not find any websites that discussed the harmful effects that starches have on the large intestine (colon), or that attribute starchy foods as a cause of human disease.

"If you consumed a lifetime supply of dairy, meat and other mucus-producing foods, you may have built up many layers of glue-like toxins on your colon walls. Although some waste can pass through your intestines daily, leading you to believe that your body is adequately digesting the food you eat, the lining of your intestines will continue to toughen and narrow." - Karyn Calabrese, *Soak Your Nuts*.

"No system of healing can be permanently effective until the eliminative organs have been thoroughly cleansed of accumulated waste matter and at the same time all grain and starchy foods have been eliminated from one's diet." – Dr. Norman W. Walker, *Become Younger*.

Let me ask you a simple question. Are you sure you want to eat that next slice of bread or bowl of rice?

Obesity

We have an obesity epidemic in this country. It is due to several factors, not all of which will be discussed in this book, but the main factors will be covered. One of the main causes for the epidemic is the consumption of saturated fats found in cooked foods, including, but not limited to, meat and dairy products and refined and processed snack foods. Because cooked foods are deficient in nutrients and enzymes, our hunger is not satisfied when we eat cooked foods, so we overeat, which compounds the problem.

It is well known that the more obese a person is, the more likely he or she will become a victim of disease. Overeating is so common in the US that it's considered "normal," even though it is a precursor of many health complications.

Overeating contributes to the wastes that build up in the body. Nutritionists, such as Dr. Robert Morse, believe that digestive juices are secreted not in proportion to the amount of food eaten, but in proportion to the amount of food that is required by the system. This may change your opinion about overeating.

As an obese person, or any other person, continues to overeat, their system becomes more and more clogged up, choked with internal undigested waste material. The resulting putrefaction causes bodily acidity and produces toxins that pollute the blood (bodily toxicity). As explained in the chapter on "The Causes of Arthritis," bodily acidity and bodily toxicity are two of the causes of arthritis.

Gluttony can cause obesity. The dictionary defines gluttony as habitual greed or excess in eating. Instead of overeating because the body senses a lack of nutrients in the foods, the glutton desires more food just for the sake of it.

From a science of nutrition point of view, gluttony may be defined as habitually eating in excess of the body's supply of gastric juices.

Overeating is so widespread that I sought additional reasons that might explain the epidemic. One of the reasons appears to be the pride or hubris that is associated with having a plentiful supply of foods. We don't face starvation in this country, just the choice between a Whopper and a Big Mac. We have more food than anyone needs or can possibly use, and in such an unrivaled variety of products. It is a supply that others in the world do not have. So, why pass up the opportunity to indulge, while you still can? Such thinking leads us into ill-health.

The dangers discussed in this chapter may be new and shocking to many readers. They were for me when I first learned about them. But they served as the impetus I needed for many of the changes I made in food selections in my diet.

Abiding by Nature's Laws

Natural laws govern our world. They include the laws of physics that encompass the mysterious forces of electromagnetism, gravity and the nuclear forces, and also the laws of biological processes, including life itself. Natural laws are always in effect, and they apply to everyone in every generation.

All creatures seem to be perfectly attuned and adjusted to these laws, except for man. We are constantly challenging or testing Nature in one way or another. Our free will, which other creatures do not have, and which sets us apart from the other creatures perhaps more than anything else, enables us to question the validity of natural laws. But Nature has a way of punishing and even eliminating people who break her laws.

In the province of Nature, things happen to us as a consequence of the way that we choose to live, the choices that we make in life, including our food choices and eating habits. For example, if I combine my foods improperly, I can expect to get a stomachache or headache. If I eat the Standard American Diet, I can expect to be the recipient of a large number of food-related health disorders that are linked to meat and dairy products and to devitalized, refined and processed foods.

The law of cause and effect is one of Nature's laws. It happens to be the foundation of the scientific method, which is the basis for all the discoveries and inventions made in the sciences, including chemistry, physics, geology, biology and the medical sciences. The law of cause and effect is observed in many clinical trials and studies that are conducted on human health and nutrition each year that show a direct relationship between the diseases of humankind and diet. Some of these trials and studies are documented in articles of the scientific and medical professions, many of which are available on the Internet, and some are cited in this book as well as in the books that are listed in the Bibliography.

If you don't want the effect, do something about the causes.

"The present ignorance of the laws underlying normal health is now, in this century, the greatest of all the past centuries, and is evidenced by the deterioration of the so-called civilized people health-wise." - Arnold Ehret, *Physical Fitness Through a Superior Diet, Fasting, and Dietetics.*

As discussed in previous chapters, many medical researchers and nutritionists claim that the cause of many human diseases are the foods that are commonly consumed, rather than normal processes of aging, such as natural "wear and tear" of the body. It is my belief that this claim will be proven to everyone's satisfaction in the years to come, impacting many popular beliefs regarding age-related health issues. An example is the degenerative disease of arthritis. Many nutritionists, including Dr. Ann Wigmore, believe that arthritis is caused by harmful dietary practices.

Raw plant foods have their enzymes intact to assist the body in their digestion, but cooking destroys food enzymes. The lack of enzymes in cooked foods causes the body to draw on its enzyme reserves for their digestion. As discussed in the last chapter, many nutritionists, such as Dr. Edward Howell, contend that this is one of the causes of degeneration in the body.

"Among the many thousands of species of creatures living on the earth, only humans and some of their domesticated animals (dogs, cats) try to live without food enzymes. And only these transgressors of nature's laws are penalized with defective health." - Dr. Edward Howell, *Enzyme Nutrition.*

The Cure for Arthritis

Fasting (simply eating less) is one of Nature's powerful ways of cleansing the body of the effects of improper diet and too much eating. When animals get sick, they instinctively abstain from food. But man seems to have lost this instinct, if he ever had it.

It is our duty to understand Nature's laws if we wish to live a healthy life, one that is free of health disorders, including diseases. The appreciation of the power of a natural law at work in us is one of the most profound things that we can ever experience.

Eating foods with their enzymes intact undestroyed by heal (raw plant foods), avoiding the dangers of cooked and starchy foods, practicing proper food combinations, and curing health issues through a combination of proper diet and fasting are only a few examples of dietary practices that adhere to the laws of Nature. You will learn about these things, and more, in this book.

Another law of nature is the need for adequate rest. In our fast-paced society, with its unrelenting demands on our time and money, our minds cry out for adequate rest. We are told that eight hours of sleep per night are required for health, but many of us get less than five. Is this abiding by Nature's laws?

"Health is the inevitable result of a strict obedience to God's physical and natural laws." - Fred S. Hirsch, *Internal Cleanliness*.

The body always lets us know how we are treating it. Understanding and heeding the warning signals the body provides helps us to maintain ourselves in concert with the laws of nature. As mentioned previously, the body can take a lot of abuse before it starts to show the ill effects of deterioration. But when that occurs, a person could be, health-wise speaking, at the point of no return.

The Cure for Arthritis

By staying proactive in this regard, we can avoid many of the health disorders, including diseases, that stalk our society.

This reveals a basic truth about our lives. The consequences of our choices are different than their effects. To avoid the perils of constipation, one must not eat foods that cause it, notwithstanding the joy one may have in doing so.

We must be concerned about the foods, the water and the air that we take into our bodies, and with the sleep and other forms of rest that we get, because they affect our chemistry and physiology for good or for bad. Moreover, we must accept Nature's laws and stop trying to alter them to meet our own desires.

"Healing is no accident. All nature heals itself when causes are removed and the conditions of health supplied." - Dr. Herbert M. Shelton.

Salt

Salt (sodium chloride) is essential to life. The Romans paid their troops in salt, hence the word "salary." Our bodies need salt, but there are different kinds of salt and some have proven to be harmful to the body.

Robert O. Young and Shelley R. Young, in their book, *The pH Miracle*, describe the differences between what they consider to be "bad salt" and "good salt." "Bad salt" is common table salt, the salt that is widely used in homes and restaurants in America and throughout the world, and is the salt that is commonly added to refined and processed foods. Let's talk about table salt before discussing the "good salt."

Nutritional experts and even members of the medical profession have implicated table salt with the high incidence of high blood pressure and kidney problems in the Western world. Table salt is unnatural, highly-refined salt that has been heat treated to very high temperatures which alters the chemical structure of the salt. The salt is then bleached white and combined with anti-caking agents, fluoride, dextrose, aluminum hydroxide (to improve its pour-ability) and preservatives. Aluminum is widely recognized as a neurotoxin and a potential cause of Alzheimer's disease. An easy way to recognize refined salt is its bleached white color.

As explained in *The pH Miracle,* many of the additives in table salt, such as those listed above, are not required to be listed on food labels, including the food labels on canned, bottled and jarred (refined and processed) foods and the food labels on packages of salt. These labels typically just list "salt" as an ingredient.

The Cure for Arthritis

The Web has some good articles about the health hazards of table salt. For example, search on "common table salt health" or "table salt poison."

F. Batmanghelidj, M.D, in his book, *Your Body's Many Cries for Salt*, states that the salt we use should be unrefined sea salt.

Jacques de Langre in his book, *Sea Salt's Hidden Powers*, states that refined and processed salt has an altered chemical structure and lacks the electrolytic positive and negative charge properties that natural sea salt possesses.

Many products with "sea salt" as an ingredient actually contain refined sea salt, not unrefined, natural sea salt. I wish I had known that years ago when I used "iodized sea salt" on my foods. *The pH Miracle* states that 89% of all sea salt commercially sold has been refined and processed, that is, its chemical structure has been altered by extreme heat and chemicals have been added. Like table salt, refined sea salt is always bleached white in color. The sea salt I was using for years was bright white in color.

Natural sea salt, the kind that comes from evaporating sea water by the heat of the sun, is not refined, meaning that it has not been heat treated by modern refining techniques, and it does not contain man-made additives. Natural sea salt has a pink or gray cast, or hue, to it; it is not bleached white.

There are several commercially available natural sea salts to choose from. An example is Celtic Sea Salt, which is North Atlantic Ocean salt. It contains over 80 minerals and is considered a full-spectrum natural sea salt. Other brands include Pink Himalayan Sea Salt and Real Salt, both of which are mined from salt deposits in the earth that apparently were formed by the Biblical Flood. Pink Himalayan sea salt comes from Pakistan. and

Real Salt comes from Utah. You can learn more about these salts on the Web.

F. Batmanghelidj in his book (referenced above) states that there are hidden "miracles" in unrefined sea salt. These include:

• Extracting excess acidity from the cells of the body, particularly the brain cells.

• Preserving the serotonin and melatonin levels in the brain.

• It is vital for the communication and information processing of nerve cells.

• Salt and water perform natural antioxidant duties and clear toxic waste from the body.

• Maintaining muscle tone and strength, reduces stress and emotional disorders and assists sleep.

"A salt-free diet is utterly stupid." - F. Batmanghelidj, *Your Body's Many Cries for Salt*.

One of the leading experts on foods and nutrition in the world today is undoubtedly David Wolfe. Some of his books are listed in the Bibliography. There is probably no one who has eaten as many different kinds of raw plant foods, or has used as many different kinds of natural sea salt, as he. For additional information about sea salt, see David Wolfe's You Tube videos on salt.

Arnold Ehret, in his book, *The Mucusless Diet Healing System*, states that salt is a very good mucus dissolver.

The Cure for Arthritis

Despite all the good that is reported about using natural sea salt, the fact remains that sea salt is an inorganic salt. Most nutritionists assert that the body cannot effectively utilize inorganic minerals of any kind, such as inorganic iodine, sodium, calcium, iron, phosphorus, magnesium, etc. They also assert that inorganic minerals not eliminated by normal bodily processes get stored in the body's tissues and joints. Nutritionists, including those referenced in this book, firmly believe that we should get all our minerals from plants.

As discussed previously, plants transform inorganic minerals from the soil and also the ocean into organic form that is easily assimilated by the body. Organic salt is contained in vegetables, including sea vegetables, and is what the body needs for health.

"The bottom line is this – no matter where or how on earth it comes from, if salt is not first transformed by plants from inorganic sodium into organic sodium, it can't be properly absorbed by the body!" - Paul C. Bragg, *Water, The Shocking Truth That Can Save Your Life*.

On a whole plant food diet. there is no lack of mineral salts for electrolyte health. If additional salt is desired because of worries about not getting enough salt, then you should use natural, unrefined sea salt.

As discussed in the chapter on "The Causes of Arthritis," Dr. Ann Wigmore healed herself of arthritis by eliminating table salt from her diet and going on a whole plant food diet.

As explained in N.W. Walker's book, *The Natural Way to Vibrant Health*, sea water has all the mineral elements in colloidal (liquid) form. He tells us how he used sea water on his foods with no adverse reactions. It appears that if water is added to natural sea salt and the salt is allowed to dissolve, it would return its minerals to colloidal form as they exist in sea water.

I have been using natural sea salt, such as Celtic Sea Salt and Real Salt, on my vegetables for years without seeing any adverse reactions such as worsening or aggravating arthritis pains. I believe that this is due to it being readily assimilated in the body.

The National Academy of Medicine (NAM) recommends limiting salt intake to 1500 mg per day, or about half a teaspoon per day.

I hope that this chapter has provided useful information regarding this important and controversial topic. If you decide to use salt, you should use natural, unrefined sea salt, and use it sparingly.

The best way to reduce our intake of refined salts is to eliminate all refined and processed foods from our diets, which includes canned, bottled and jarred foods, packaged refined and processed snack foods, and fast foods. Another way is to be a smart shopper and check the ingredients for salt before you buy food products, including condiments, that contain large quantities of salt, such as mustard and ketchup.

The Cure for Arthritis

Distilled Water

"Pure distilled water is truly God's greatest gift to us, a source of life and health." - Paul C. Bragg.

Drinking distilled water has received a bad rap over the years. This chapter explains why distilled water is, in fact, beneficial to human health and should be the water of choice for all who strive for optimum health.

Contrary to popular belief/misconception, our blood is not comprised of regular water. Human blood is comprised of about 78% fluid, and 90% of it is distilled water. According to nutritional experts, including Dr. N. W. Walker, Paul C. Bragg, and Dr. Allen E. Banik (who spent most of his life researching the effects of water on the human body), we do not need regular water to sustain health, and, more significantly, regular water is harmful to human health. This startling contention is explored in this chapter.

As we progress in our understanding of foods and nutrition, many of the things that humankind has taken for granted throughout the centuries may be exposed as untruths or falsehoods.

Regular water, which includes tap or faucet water, drinking-fountain water, spring, well, river and lake water, is water that has been in contact with rocks and soil. It also includes filtered water since most minerals in regular water are in solution[31] and do not get filtered out. What we normally refer to as "water" includes all of the aforementioned types. They contain inorganic minerals, such as lime (calcium), sodium, iron, phosphorus, magnesium,

---

[31] The most commonly dissolved minerals are sodium, calcium, magnesium, potassium, chloride, bicarbonate and sulfate.

etc., that have been collected from the rocks or soil that the water has been in contact with.

Distilled water has no inorganic minerals and is devoid of chlorination and fluoridation, heavy metals and pesticides. It is the type of water most compatible with the human body's cells. It is entirely safe for human consumption, and ideally meets the needs of the body.

Also, contrary to popular belief/misconception, distilled water does not leach out minerals that have become part of the body's cells. This in confirmed in Robert Morse's book, *The Detox Miracle Sourcebook*, which states that distilled water dissolves inorganic minerals that are lodged in the tissues and joints of the body, and greatly assists in removing them from the body, but it does not cause minerals that are part of the body's cells to be leached out.

Dr. N. W. Walker in his book, *Water Can Undermine Your Health*, states the following:

"It is virtually impossible for distilled water to separate minerals which have become an integral part of the cells and tissues of the body. Distilled water collects only the minerals which remain in the body, minerals discarded from natural water and from the cells, the minerals which the natural water originally collected from its contact with the earth and the rocks. Such minerals, having been rejected by the cells of the body are of no constructive value. On the contrary, they are debris which distilled water is capable of picking up and eliminating from the system." - Dr. N. W. Walker, *Water Can Undermine Your Health*.

Again, distilled water cannot leach out minerals that have become part of the body's cells. What it can do is leach out excess minerals that are deposited in the joints and tissues of the body, minerals that the body could not properly utilize.

"Distilled water acts as a solvent in the body. It dissolves food substances so they can be assimilated and taken into every cell. It dissolves inorganic mineral substances lodged in tissues of the body so that such substances can be eliminated in the process of purifying the body. Distilled water is the greatest solvent on earth, the only one that can be taken into the body without damage to the tissues. By its continued use, it is possible to dissolve inorganic minerals, acid crystals, and all the other waste products of the body without injuring tissues." - Dr. Allen E. Banik, *The Choice is Clear*.

Organic minerals are the minerals we get from eating plants. Plants convert the inorganic minerals found in the water that they take up from the soil into a readily usable-by-the-body organic form. Organic minerals are not deposited in the tissues and joints of the body but are utilized by the cells for their regeneration.

Distilled water is regular, hard water that has been condensed after the water is boiled. Distillation is the most effective method of purifying water. The minerals stay behind because they are not volatile, and the condensed steam is pure of minerals, bacteria, viruses and physical impurities. Even rain water is not as pure as distilled water since it contains impurities picked up by the rain from the air.

Since the time that municipal water was first chlorinated, it has been maintained by many that drinking regular water, the water that originates from streams and lakes, which includes municipal recycled water, mineral waters and bottled waters, is good for health because it has minerals the body needs. However, according to many nutritionists, inorganic minerals that are contained in regular water should not be put into the human body.

"There is only one way you can purify your body and help to eliminate your chronic aging diseases and that is through the miracle of distilled water." - Dr. Allen E. Banik, *The Choice is Clear.*

In addition to lacking inorganic minerals, distilled water is totally lacking in dangerous metals and chemicals that are found in today's drinking and bottled waters.

Paul and Patricia Bragg, in their book *Water, The Shocking Truth That Can Change Your Life*, state that the tap water we use for cooking, bathing and drinking can be responsible for many ailments because of the addition of harmful chemicals such as sodium fluoride and chlorine. The book explains the dangers of these chemicals. The authors further state that distilled water is the only water we should drink, not only because it removes inorganic mineral deposits and toxins from the joints of the body, but because it helps remove cholesterol and fat.

"Inorganic minerals, toxic chemicals, fluoride and contaminants can pollute, clog up and even turn tissues to stone throughout your body, causing pain, illness and even premature death!" - Paul C. Bragg, *Water, The Shocking Truth That Can Save Your Life*.

For similar reasons, Dr. N. W. Walker, in his many books, states that distilled water should be used for cooking and drinking.

"Distilled water is always the safest to drink. As regular water may leave deposits of calcium and other unwanted minerals in the blood circulation, these may find their way into the endocrine gland system with disastrous results which might never be attributed to these unusable minerals as the cause." - Norman W. Walker, *Water Can Undermine Your Health*.

Some people have purchased reverse osmosis water filtration units for under-the-sink home use to purify their faucet water for drinking or cooking purposes. In the reverse osmosis process, water is purified by forcing a portion of the faucet water through a semi-permeable membrane. The process removes a high percentage of the dissolved solids as well as other contaminants from the water. However, Dr. Allen E. Banik, in his book, *The Choice is Clear*, explains why reverse osmosis water is not preferable to distilled water, in the following excerpt:

"While the result [of reverse osmosis] often approaches the purity of distilled water. the degree of purity in any case varies widely, depending on the types and conditions of the equipment used, much as with filter equipment, and the effectiveness lessens with use, sometimes drastically!" - Dr. Allen E. Banik, *The Choice is Clear*.

The advantages of drinking distilled water are many as described above. From my researching, I did not find any disadvantages except for what appears on websites. For the websites that were polled for this information, I did not find any that supported the claims of the nutritionists that have been cited in this chapter. Once again, this exemplifies the disconnect that exists between the truths about foods and nutrition versus the claims on popular media.

I have been drinking distilled water for years with absolutely no ill effects. I switched from hard, faucet and bottle waters to distilled water when I read the books that describe the health benefits of drinking distilled water. I find its taste to be much better than faucet water or bottled waters, and I can testify to the positive difference it makes in my health.

The Cure for Arthritis

My recommendation is that everyone on the raw vegan diet switch to drinking distilled water for their health. The next time you are shopping for bottled water, pick up a gallon of distilled water instead. At the time of this writing, distilled water was selling for about eighty cents per gallon at retail stores like Wal-Mart.

Within the first month of drinking distilled water, I noticed a marked increase in my thirst for the water. Previously, it seemed that I never drank very much water and I never liked the taste of it when I drank it. But now, I love the taste of water in its purist form, with its thirst-quenching ability as a bonus. Distilled water is, for me, a truly rewarding experience. There is something about distilled water and the actions it performs on the body that are very remarkable. Distilled water is what I believe the body craves.

It is said that the older we get the more we lose our ability to sense thirst. As a result, our bodies become more and more dehydrated as we continue to age, without us being able to recognize it. This chronic dehydration can cause serious health problems.

"Chronic and persistently increasing dehydration is the root cause of almost all currently encountered diseases of the human body." - F. Batmanghelidj, M.D, *Your Body's Many Cries for Water*.

What has changed my life more than anything else in recent years has been switching to the raw vegan diet and drinking distilled water.

Guidelines that Don't Work and Laws that Do

The United States Department of Agriculture (USDA) has issued its Food Guide Pyramid since 1992. The Guide is intended to help Americans reduce their intake of total fat and choose what and how much to eat from each of the food groups that are depicted on the pyramid. The government's involvement in the issuance of nutritional guidelines shows how far we have drifted away from the basics of proper health and nutrition.

The food pyramid is often displayed on packaged foods, such as breads. However, it is the firm conviction of many of nutritionists that the USDA Food Pyramid does not, and never has, properly reflected what is best for human health. Rather, it reflects what the food industry says is best for health.

The meat, dairy and grain businesses, which are the chief vested interests in perpetuating the Standard American Diet, have influenced federal dietary regulations for decades. It is commonly believed that these interests write the protocols of the USDA. As stated in a dietary guideline article published on the Web, "After all, what is the USDA if not the regulatory body created to ensure that the U.S. agricultural commodities (like corn, soy, and wheat) are profitable?" These interests are interested first, last and always in profits, not in human welfare.

It is well known that most of the grain produced in the world goes to feed livestock in order to supply food stores and restaurants with cold cuts and other meat products.

Most of us realize by now the power that big businesses have to make the rules. But health awareness and a knowledge of foods

The Cure for Arthritis

and nutrition give us the freedom to eat the healthier foods that are available for us to eat.

The food pyramid is not our friend. When I started searching for the answers about how foods and nutrition impact human health years ago, I was often led astray by the food pyramid because of my gullibility to accept what governmental bodies recommend should be my diet. As discussed in this book, many nutritionists, including those whose books are listed in the Bibliography, have been telling us for years that meat, dairy and grain products are harmful to human health.

The food pyramid of 1992 to 2005 (see below) shows bread, cereal, rice and pasta at the bottom, or base, of the pyramid, indicating that grain products should be the most often eaten food. However, all grains, even raw grain seeds, are starchy foods. And pasta, sweet rolls and bread are cooked foods. As discussed in this book, cooked and starchy foods are harmful to human health. For a healthy diet, the food pyramid would not have grain products as the base, nor would it include cooked foods.

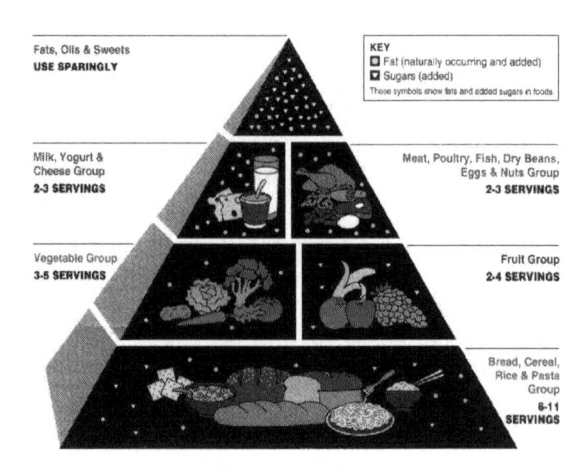

The Food Guide Pyramid from 1992 to 2005

The Cure for Arthritis

The food pyramid of 2005 to 2011 (below), makes even less sense. It doesn't have a clearly defined base or hierarchy. It shows five food groups (grains, vegetables, fruits, milk, and meat and beans), sharing the same base. There is no one food group at the base of the pyramid. At first glance, it indicates that there is no one food group any better for health than another. It implies that you should eat a portion of each.

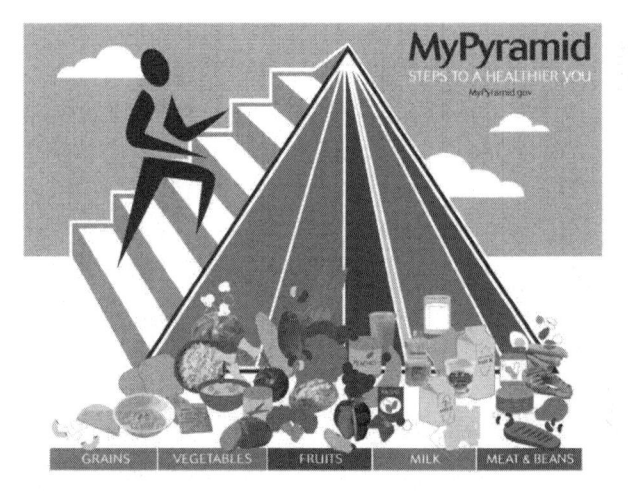

The Food Guide Pyramid from 2005 to 2011

It is not surprising that grains, milk and meat are three of the five food groups that share the base of this food pyramid. The meat, dairy and grain businesses are those with the largest vested interests in continuing the production of animal products for the Standard American Diet.

For most of us, the food pyramid of 2005 to 2011 is too confusing to be an effective dietary guideline.

The Food Pyramid has recently (2019) been superseded by MyPlate (see below), also published by the USDA. MyPlate is a

The Cure for Arthritis

depiction of a pie-shaped plate of food on a table with a drink off to one side. Five food groups, Fruits, Vegetables, Grains, Proteins and Milk, are represented.

There are no MyPlate details in the depiction to reveal what each food group consists of, but they may be accessed on the Web. For example, for Fruits, the details list as options, fresh, canned, frozen, dried, cut up or pureed. For Proteins, the details list seafood, meat, poultry and eggs, nuts, seeds and soy. The drink off to the side is milk. The dangers of eating canned food products, and most of the protein options (excepting nuts and seeds), have been discussed in this book. Also, as discussed previously, vegetables provide all the protein needed for human health. The MyPlate design implies that we need to eat foods from all five food groups, including dairy, and in every form sold to the public.

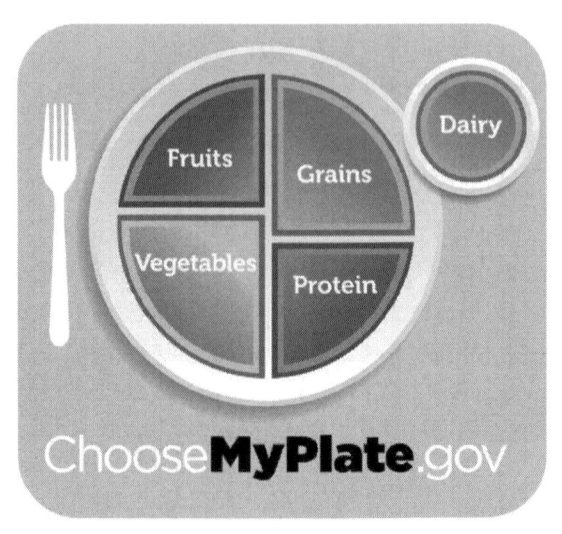

The current (2019) USDA Food Guideline

The Cure for Arthritis

In the age of information, a food pyramid or pie plate that would really make sense would be one that would give priority to eating raw fruits and vegetables over everything else, with nuts, seeds, and water included in the design. It would not include meat- and dairy-based foods, grain products or canned foods.

However, it probably doesn't matter what the food pyramids or other depictions look like. Guidelines do not make people knowledgeable no matter how instructive they may be. Knowledge about foods and nutrition is not gained by glancing at a food pyramid or pie chart. Our current obesity epidemic, as described in the chapter on "Dangers to Avoid," clearly indicates the public's failure to follow any dietary guidelines.

People make society what it is. Most people eat whatever they want as often as they want, regardless of the complications and discomforts that result. But what most people eat and how they eat does not have to be the way that we eat.

Each of us can work to produce a better society by the food choices we make every day. As mentioned previously, unless we have a knowledge of foods and nutrition, we lack the information needed on how health issues come about. Without this knowledge, we remain wholly ignorant of how to prevent diseases and other health disorders from taking root in the soil of the body, and how to cure them if they do. A knowledge of foods and nutrition enables us to make the right food choices, those that result in real health, which is health in tune with Nature.

Proper Food Combinations

"Cook not, neither mix all things one with another, lest your bowels become as steaming bogs...for I tell you truly, if you mix together all sorts of food in your body, then the peace of your body will cease, and endless war will rage in you." - Attributed to Jesus, *The Essene Gospel of Peace, Book One.*

Before food can nourish the body, it must be digested. Digestion is a chemical process that breaks down food into constituents that can be assimilated by the body. Digestion starts in the mouth with saliva and continues in the stomach where digestive juices, or gastric juices, are secreted to break down the food. The job of digestion is not finished until the food travels through the small and large intestines and the wastes pass out of the body.

Food combination laws are rules of nature that are based on the principle that different types of foods require different times for digestion, and cause the secretion in the stomach of different types of gastric juices, some being more acidic, some less acidic. If we eat foods that cause more alkaline (less acidic) gastric juices for their digestion together with foods that require more acidic juices for their digestion, the juices combine, resulting in food in the stomach that is difficult to digest. This leads to a variety of complications, such as stomachaches, headaches and fermentation, and, when the food passes through the intestines, putrefaction, gas and the breeding of parasites.

When foods are difficult to digest, the energy reserves of the body are called into play to assist in the job of digestion. It should not be surprising that you feel tired after eating a big meal of improperly combined foods -- the traditional nap after a Thanksgiving dinner.

The stomach does not decide what foods to put in it. It leaves that job to the brain.

The Web adequately covers many aspects of proper food combining. A good website on proper food combining at the time of this writing is: https: //www.acidalkalinediet.net/correct-food-combining-principles.php.

However, some Web articles on food combining do not stand up to careful scrutiny. For example, some tell us that combining nuts with sweet fruits is an improper food combination. But based on my experience, and what nutritional experts tell us, fatty nuts (like walnuts and pecans) combine well with some sweet fruits, such as bananas and dates. Other sweet fruits, such as apples; that have a high water content, make the nuts indigestible.

In *The Sunfood Diet Success System*, David Wolfe explains that nuts are actually fat-dominant, not protein-dominant, foods because they consist mostly of fat. He explains that the fat in nuts and seeds allows the natural sugar in sweet fruit to be time-released, which helps digestion and provides more long-term energy. Combining sweet fruits with fatty nuts and seeds is an acceptable food combination, contrary to some of the articles on the Web.

The food combination laws should be learned, even if one or two of them are not correctly stated on the Web. The laws that are not correctly stated on the Web at least err on the safe side so that by observing them you will not be hurting yourself. Set goals for yourself to rigidly put the laws into practice.

The rules of food combining are soundly rooted in physiology and thoroughly tested by experience.

"More than sixty years spent in feeding the well and the sick, the weak and the strong, the old and the young, have demonstrated that a change to correctly combined meals is followed by an immediate improvement in health as a consequence of lightening the load the digestive organs have to carry, thus assuring better digestion." - Herbert M. Shelton, *Food Combining Made Easy*.

I enjoy many foods by themselves, but I'm an inveterate mixer. I prefer to mix my foods, to combine them. I learned the food combination laws the hard way, by trial and error, and suffered all the resulting stomachaches of improperly combined foods. Very probably, you will learn them the hard way too. It took me about a year to put the laws into practice without making further mistakes.

Five of the food combination laws that are important on any diet, including the raw vegan diet, are as follows.

1. Don't Eat Proteins with Starches

Example: Spirulina or hemp seed (both protein foods) eaten with Maca (a starchy food).

2. Don't Eat Starches with Acid Fruit

Example: Potatoes or peas (both starchy foods) eaten with tomatoes (acid fruit).

Note that tomatoes combine well with leafy greens and fatty plant foods like avocados.

3. Don't Eat Starches with Sweet or Sub-Acid Fruit

Example: Beans or peas (starchy foods) added to green smoothies that contain sweet or sub-acid fruit.

I have my own rule for this – don't add vegetables other than leafy greens to green smoothies. I've had too many stomachaches from breaking this law, so I make it easier to remember by excluding all vegetables (except greens) from my green smoothies which contain sweet fruit.

4. Don't Eat Sweet Fruit with Acid Fruit

Example: Pineapple (an acid fruit) eaten with bananas or dates (sweet fruit).

Note that sweet fruit combines well with sub-acid fruits, such as apricots.

5. Don't Eat Proteins with Sweet Fruit

Example: Hemp seed with dates. Hemp seed is 30% protein. Higher protein foods, such as spirulina, are even worse combinations with sweet fruit because they cause severe gas resulting from the fermentation that occurs. Bananas are an exception because they combine well with nuts and seeds.

The above food combination laws cover some of the errors typically made on the raw vegan diet. Additional food combination laws should also be learned. As explained previously, you can learn about them on the Web.

Greens (green leafy vegetables) are the only foods that combine well with all other foods, including other greens.

To aid in preparing meals, the digestion times required for different types of foods should also be learned. Obviously, we should not combine foods that require completely different digestion times. Digestion times for different foods are adequately covered on the Web. Typically, digestion times and proper food combinations go hand in hand.

When the food combination laws are obeyed, digestion is greatly improved and overall well-being is enhanced. When food combination laws are broken, stomachaches, headaches, excessive flatulence, or other complications can and do result, which can quickly turn what started out to be a good day into a bad one.

"Improved digestion results in general improvement in all the functions of life. Many and great are the benefits to flow from improved digestion." - Dr. Herbert M. Shelton, *Food Combining Made Easy.*

How to Determine the Starch Content of Foods

Food labels (Nutrition Facts Labels) typically give the amount of total carbohydrates, sugar and fiber, but not the amount of starch in the food. The starch content might be published on the Web, but if it's not, here's how to determine the starch content of any food from its Nutrition Facts Label.

From the food label on the product package, or as given on the Web, get the weights in grams of total carbohydrates, sugars and fiber and plug them into the following equation:

Starch = Carbs – (Sugars + Fiber).

Example 1: Maca. On the Web, the Nutrition Facts Label for Maca lists, for a 100g serving: 71g carbs, 32g sugars and 7g fiber.

Starch (g) = 71g – (32g + 7g) = 71g – 39g = 32g

32g/100g = 32%

The Cure for Arthritis

Maca is 32% starch. Since starch content is a considerable portion of Maca, it is a starchy vegetable.

<u>Example 2</u>: Carrots. Per the Web, a 61g serving of carrots has 6g carbs, 2.9g sugars and 1.7g fiber.

Starch (g) = 6g – (2.9g + 1.7g) = 6g – 4.8g = 1.2g

1.2g/61g = 2%

Carrots are 2% starch. Since the starch content of carrots is very low, it is a non-starchy vegetable.

Many articles on the Web differ on whether carrots are starchy or non-starchy vegetables. Some articles say carrots are starchy vegetables while others say they are non-starchy vegetables. This is another example of conflicting information found on the Web.

<u>Example 3</u>: Beets. Per the Web, a 100g serving of beets has 10g carbs, 7g sugars and 2.8g fiber.

Similar to the above computations, beets are 0.2% starch. It is a non-starchy vegetable.

<u>Example 4</u>: Turnips. Per the Web, a 122g serving of turnips has 8g carbs, 4.6g sugars and 2.2g fiber.

Similar to the above computations, turnips are 0.1% starch. It is a non-starchy vegetable.

<u>Example 5</u>: Cinnamon. Per the Web, a 7.8g serving of cinnamon has: 6g carbs, 4.1g sugars and 0.2g fiber.

Similar to the above computations, cinnamon is 21% starch. Cinnamon is a starchy food. It should not be used with protein foods or with sweet or sub-acid fruit.

As the proper combination of hydrocarbons in your vehicle's fuel determines how it runs, so your life will run smoothly if your foods are eaten in their proper combinations. In my opinion, if positive feedback is not received by the body on any food that is eaten, no matter what the type or variety -- fruit, vegetable, Superfood, herb or any other kind of food -- then that food should either be eaten in a more ripe condition, in smaller quantities, in proper combinations with other foods, or it should be avoided. The body is no fool. It recognizes foods that disagree with it or do it harm by giving us warning signals. Our job then is to correctly interpret these signals.

The Blood

"The life of the flesh is in the blood." - Lev. 17:11.

This chapter describes the effects that foods have on blood health and shows how to interpret your own blood condition.

Blood is life. As the poets claim, it is the song of the lark, the blush on the cheek, the spring of the lamb. It is the sacred wine in the silver chalice. Down through the ages, blood has been the price men paid for freedom, and so it is today. Blood is our most preciously guarded possession.

Nutritionists tell us that the quality of the blood starts changing within a few hours after eating a meal. Blood cells, like other cells of the body, are continually being replaced. Old cells are being replaced by new cells. The new cells are constructed from the raw materials that foods and drinks provide. The quality of the blood depends a great deal on the quality of the foods that are eaten. When we eat cooked foods, including refined and processed foods, blood cells are constructed of inferior-quality building materials, materials that are devoid of the life force properties that raw plant foods possess.

"Dead atoms and dead molecules cannot rejuvenate or re-generate the cells of the body. Such food results in cell starvation and this in turn causes sickness and disease." – Dr. Norman W. Walker, *Water Can Undermine Your Health*.

As discussed in the chapter on "The Causes of Arthritis," acidity is a blood condition mainly brought on by eating too many acid-producing foods. When we eat foods typical of a cooked meat and/or pasteurized milk diet, which are acidic foods, the blood becomes thick and heavy which causes clogging in the tissues and is known to adversely affect the arteries and lymphatic system, and cause poor circulation and elevated blood pressure. When we eat whole plant foods such as raw fruits, vegetables and leafy greens, the blood's condition becomes normal, which is alkaline, and is not thickened which results in improved circulation and reduced blood pressure.

"Animal foods cannot build good blood; in fact, do not build human blood at all, because of the biological fact that man is by nature a fruit eater. Look at the juice of a ripe blackberry, black cherry or black grapes. Doesn't it almost resemble your blood? Can any reasonable man prove that half-decayed "muscle tissue" builds better blood?" - Arnold Ehret, *Mucusless Diet Healing System*.

Berg's Tables, provided in Appendix I, list common foods that are "acid-forming" or "acid-binding". According to the tables, meat and grain products are the most acid-forming foods, whereas fruits and vegetables are the most acid-binding foods.

Almost all raw plant foods are alkaline, or become alkaline in the body. Fruits of the Citrus genus (oranges, grapefruit, etc.) are alkalizing in the body despite their initial acidity. If we ate nothing but raw fruits, leafy greens and vegetables, our blood chemistry would be alkaline most of the time. The times when it would not be so would be in times of stress, or when we are exposed to environmental toxins, or are taking alcohol, caffeine or medication. Grains, most legumes, and most commonly eaten nuts are acid-forming (and mucus-forming) foods to some extent.

The chlorophyll in leafy green vegetables cleanses and alkalizes the blood. The body converts chlorophyll into heme, an iron compound that is part of hemoglobin, to produce red blood cells. Unfortunately, many Americans do not eat greens except in small

The Cure for Arthritis

amounts, such as lettuce in fast food sandwiches, which is one of the reasons why many people in this country are lacking in vitamins, antioxidants, and the therapeutic properties that plant foods have. Greens include spinach, kale, chard, lettuces, cabbages, collard greens and mustard greens. The importance of eating greens for health is discussed throughout this book.

As discussed in the chapter on "The Causes of Arthritis," homeostasis is the tendency of the body to maintain itself in stable chemical equilibrium. Health is said to be a balancing act with the body trying to balance or stabilize itself to a normal or alkaline blood condition. Obviously, the effectiveness at doing this is encumbered or enhanced by the foods that are eaten, and how they are eaten. An acidic blood condition is typically caused by a nutrient deficient diet. If the diet is continued, the blood condition worsens to where the body's attempts at homeostasis are not sufficient in neutralizing the acidic condition. The acids the body cannot neutralize and expel as waste get stored in the tissues and joints of the body which can lead to diseases.

Two examples of the effects of a poor blood condition are anemia, a condition of not having enough healthy red blood cells, and deep-vein thrombosis, which is blood clotting. Healthy blood does not produce these disorders.

According to Dr. Michael Greger's book, *How Not To Die*, plant-based diets have been shown to reduce the risk of blood cancers by 50%.

pH Balance

Nature's way is for the human body to maintain its blood in an alkaline pH range of 7.35 - 7.45, the range that the body tries to maintain at all times through the process of homeostasis. pH is a term used in chemistry for the amount of acidity or alkalinity of an aqueous solution. The pH scale runs from 0 to 14, with a pH of 7 being neutral, a pH of less than 7 being acidic, and a pH greater than 7 being alkaline.

The basal pH of gastric juices secreted by the glands of the stomach is strongly acidic, with a range of 1.5 - 3.5. The pH in the stomach changes when food is in the stomach, and is influenced by a number of psychological factors, including the aroma and taste of foods.

Blood Sampling and Analysis

A blood test is often prescribed by doctors to help diagnose a person's health condition. The blood sample is sent to a laboratory where technicians analyze the blood using specialized instruments and techniques. Various tests may be performed on a blood sample, including a complete blood count (CBC), which is used to detect a wide range of health disorders such as anemia, infection and leukemia, and a blood glucose test which is used to help diagnose diabetes and monitor blood glucose levels. None of the tests are conclusive in themselves but are used to help diagnose a patient's condition and determine what follow-up tests should be prescribed.

In Appendix D of his book, *The Detox Miracle Sourcebook*, Robert Morse describes how anyone can interpret the results of the blood work that a doctor has prescribed for them. It includes a description of blood types (Types A, B, AB, etc.), the meaning of red and white blood cell counts, and the limitations that the diagnostics have. It lists reference ranges for nutrients that are found in the blood. The ranges are based on analyses of blood of presumably healthy people. But the point is, it seems that the body requires nutrients to be within certain ranges for health.

The Cure for Arthritis

According to T. Colin Campbell in his book, *Whole, Rethinking the Science of Nutrition*, the body is continually monitoring and adjusting the concentrations of nutrients in the blood to maintain the ranges it requires for health. He explains how medical and governmental understanding of nutrition is rooted in the *reductionist paradigm*, a way of thinking that everything can be understood through its component parts. He contends that a wholistic approach to health is what is required to understand nutrition. A wholistic approach considers how the various component parts work together, which is in line with how nature operates. Nature works in wholistic ways, with all parts working together, never with one part working on its own. This is a very important concept to understand in our journey to optimum health.

"When you're looking through a microscope, either literally or metaphorically, you can't see the big picture." - T. Colin Campbell and Howard Jacobson, *Whole, Rethinking the Science of Nutrition*.

An old saying seems to be apropos here, "You can't see the forest for the trees." We cannot see the forest when we are focusing on the trees.

Nutritionists have known for many years that the condition of the urine reveals much about the blood's condition. For example, if the urine is cloudy, the blood is likely to be cloudy too, such as when protein intake has thickened it. The pH of urine closely matches the pH of the blood, and can be used to determine the blood's pH condition. Litmus paper is a useful tool in this regard. It is another example of how we can become more our own doctor. We can test our urine's pH. Strips of litmus paper may be purchased on the Web.

More on how to be your own doctor is covered in the next chapter.

How to Be Your Own Doctor

The cure for arthritis starts with the clear realization that we can do something about our health issues ourselves. After all, it is our responsibility to take care of our bodies. It is not our doctor's, our spouse's, our friends' or the Government's; it is our responsibility.

The best way to reach health goals is to take charge of your own health and learn how to be your own doctor. Nobody is born with knowledge; it must be gained. When the knowledge required to promote and sustain health is gained and put into practice, practically any health issue that assails us can be effectively dealt with without the doctors' advice. It equips us to become, in many ways, our own doctors. This reality has far reaching consequences for our health and well-being, providing numerous health benefits, and preventing numerous health disorders.

The more we learn about foods and nutrition, how to detoxify the body, how to properly combine foods, etc., the more we become our own doctors. It is then that we can resolve our own health issues, and often in ways that completely surprise us. One day they're there, and a few days later they're gone. It is all due to the amazing powers of living plant foods to cleanse the body of its impurities and restore us to health.

Ordinary diets, chaotic and haphazard food combining and unhealthy food cravings produce sickness. But a diet of life-giving foods, and the other practices that are described in this book enable the body to heal itself of practically any health disorder, including cancer, heart disease and the many lesser ailments of which humankind is susceptible.

The Cure for Arthritis

The process proceeds something like this. Health improvements begin with the realization that a healthy diet must be embraced, which is gained by a knowledge of foods and nutrition. Then comes the somewhat harder part, putting into practice what has been learned. But it gets easier as we experience health improvements as the body rids itself of accumulated toxins and we fine-tune our diet based on feedback from the body.

The body is much wiser than we may think it is. It affects the mind so significantly that it may be said to control the mind. Eating a whole plant food diet results in genuine health, which profoundly affects the mind by increasing mental stamina and clarity.

The health corner is turned when we give up foods that are harmful to the body and eat foods that promote health. There is something about eating raw plant foods that strikes a chord of recognition deep within us, as though we intuitively know that these foods are best for us.

Although some people see health improvement from eating whole plant foods in a relatively short time, one should not expect to reverse a lifetime of improper eating habits overnight, or in a matter of days or weeks. But if you have the willpower to change, health improvements will occur. But bear in mind, as stated earlier, that no cure can be expected to work while harmful eating habits and food cravings are constantly counteracting the cure.

"Nature takes her time to heal and cure, but the results are lasting. When people appreciate this, and try it, they learn that Nature wants man to live a life of simplicity. It is man who makes life complicated." - Dr. Norman W. Walker.

Since health conditions are quickly resolved on a whole plant food diet, the time and money saved on doctors and prescriptions can be used for other things. Energy levels increase and health cares no longer burden us.

Being your own doctor has advantages besides saving money on hospital stays and doctor bills. The sense of accomplishment and the boost in self-esteem that follows being able to heal yourself of a health issue are priceless rewards. Is there a doctor in the house? Yes, and it's you!

What is better for the budget than raw fruits and vegetables? When we purchase refined and processed foods, we are paying a premium for what was done to them. In comparison, natural foods are much less expensive. Local food stores typically sell onions for under a dollar a pound, and a large cluster of garlic cloves for about half a dollar. Onions and garlic are marvelous foods, and do not have to be purchased organic. A large bunch of carrots, two heads of cabbage, a head of cauliflower, several onions, a cluster of celery, some lemons and a bunch of bananas typically costs less than 10 USD, and may last for more than a week.

Many people do not realize how their health influences their feelings about life. If you wake up feeling groggy, sluggish and in a sour mood, you may not know why but the cause very likely lies within. It is probably due to the accumulated toxins and waste matter that reside within you, not only in the colon but in the very tissues of your body, toxins that have not yet been purged by the body's self-cleansing process. The biological disharmony that this creates is most evident first thing in the morning.

The disharmony felt in the mornings can be caused by what we ate the day before or the night before, or by how we ate it. A way of life discordant with the laws of nature destroys the harmony of the organism. Likewise, a way of life in harmony with her laws preserves the harmony of the organism.

Stay with the diet and you will reap the benefits of it. Give up during times of disappointment or frustration, and all will be lost.

Remember that if the attainment of genuine health required no knowledge or effort or discernment whatsoever on the part of an individual, then everyone would be remarkably healthy.

Being our own doctor in essence means learning all we can about foods and nutrition from informed sources, such as the books that are referenced in the Bibliography, then putting into practice what is learned and heeding the signals the body gives us about the foods and substances we ingest.

"Life's greatest achievement is the continual remaking of yourself so that at last you know how to live." - Winfred Rhodes.

Natural cures have one thing in common, they aim at correcting the underlying causes of health issues instead of suppressing their symptoms.

How Eating Habits are Formed

Let's start with the basics. I have often found it beneficial to examine the things that are taken for granted, especially when it comes to foods and nutrition.

Whether young or old, male or female, the main criterion for food choices for most people is how foods taste and go down rather than how they affect health. In other words, taste-appeal over health-appeal. Unfortunately, this truth has been exploited by the many concerns of the food industry in the creation of many substances that are added to our foods and drinks to make them more appetizing.

The Cure for Arthritis

The second basis for food selection is the emotional pulls that certain foods have on us. Both of these food selection reasons drive the majority of our decisions about foods. They also cause food habits to form.

Food habits are long-standing patterns of behavior associated with eating. Those of us who grew up on burgers, French fries and soft drinks tend to stick with that menu, or slight variations of it, throughout life, unless of course change is initiated.

It is now evident to most people that many of the health disorders prevalent in this country and throughout the world are diet-related. However, as stated previously, many of us continue to eat just as we did last year and the year before because of our habits. Another reason is that we have been culturally indoctrinated to believe that certain foods, such as meat and dairy products, sugary foods and drinks, and refined and processed foods, are good for us. Both pressures are reducing our numbers rapidly. Eating foods that we grew up on is not working.

A habit once formed and persistently practiced eventually turns into a craving, whether for chocolates, ice cream, sweet rolls or anything else. The worst part of cravings is that they stay with us even when they are doing us harm. Food cravings are encouraged by the many advertisements in the media for foods and drinks. Despite their oftentimes silky persuasiveness, the products being sold are, for the most part, refined and processed foods and drinks that have been heat treated, chemically altered, devitalized and robbed of precious nutrients. Not surprisingly, many of the ads support the meat, dairy and grain interests, the chief vested interests in our food industry.

But anyone with a little persistence and willpower can change their eating habits. Healthy eating habits are formed when we become convinced that dietary change is in our best interests.

As stated previously, by choosing to ignore the information that has been gained in the human health field which proves that diseases and a host of lesser human ailments are caused by commonly eaten foods, many of us are sacrificing our health for eating habits and food cravings. But the remarkable truth is that eating habits can be changed, even when food cravings exist, and that everyone is capable of changing their diet in enlightened self-interest.

<u>Proper Eating Habits</u>

"We are not what we eat but what we assimilate" - Paavo O. Airola.

Those who wolf, gulp or bolt down their foods are prone to digestive discomforts and disorders, including heartburn and stomachache to mention only two. Many regularly resort to quick remedies, such as antacids, aspirin and similar drugs. According to the Web, at least $2 billion is spent yearly in the US alone on antacids, and $10 billion worldwide. That's a lot of indigestion!

In addition, many people eat compulsively, often consuming food throughout the day whenever they feel like it, whether they're hungry or not. Compulsive eating can be out of habit or because of job-prescribed or tradition-prescribed meal times. If we eat food when we are not hungry, the body is not ready for the food.

These habits are damaging to the human system, and the damage gets worse the more they are practiced. They cannot produce vibrant health because the foods cannot be properly digested and assimilated by the body. Not only do they cause digestive difficulties, but they cause sluggishness and grogginess, general fatigue and various illnesses. An old saying is:

One quarter of what you eat keeps you alive. The other quarter keeps your doctor alive.

Proper eating habits are prescribed by Nature. Food must be eaten in such a way that the full powers of the digestive system are employed. In addition, every ounce of food that passes through the body that is not actually needed by the body is a tax on the body's vital powers, a waste of vital energy.

To avoid these complications and more, most of us need to modify our eating habits.

Digestion occurs primarily in two ways, mechanical digestion and chemical digestion.

Mechanical digestion occurs as the teeth grind and masticate foods. Chewing breaks down food into smaller particles which allows them to be better digested. An old saying is: *Chew your food, your stomach has no teeth.*

Chemical digestion begins in the mouth through saliva. The process of chewing activates the flow of saliva. If the mouth does not water during a meal then the body is not ready for the food, and digestion of that food will be hindered. Some nutritionists claim that food well-salivated is practically half-digested before it gets to the stomach. Many raw foodists recommend chewing food until it is liquified in the mouth. In addition, when whole plant foods are eaten, the enzymes in these foods assist in the chemical digestive process.

The Cure for Arthritis

Two thousand years ago, Asclepiades of Greece understood that particles of food are a main cause of indigestion. If the particles were small, digestion would follow its normal course, but if the particles were too big, indigestion would occur.

"The chief function of today's cook is to prepare soft pap for the adult, so that little or no chewing is required. Meats are pounded or ground and vegetables cooked to make them easy to swallow with a minimum of chewing; breads are made to be swallowed with very little preliminary mastication; potatoes are mashed, cereals soaked and fruits stewed, so that the muscles of the jaw get very little exercise and the food gets very little saliva. There is no real pleasure in such eating." - Dr. Herbert M. Shelton, *Health for the Millions.*

To get the most out of foods, and produce the kind of health we all want and need, the following eating habits should be practiced at every meal.

1. All foods should be eaten slowly, and chewed thoroughly. If you are very hungry before eating, you should still slow down on the eating or the foods will be wolfed or bolted down with little chewing taking place.

2. Do not overeat. This is the cardinal rule to master if you want to obtain optimum health. The best advice I can offer is the same as that of many others, which is to leave the table when you are 2/3 full. This has often been difficult for me to learn, but I found that when I practiced it everything changed for the better on my journey to optimum health. What it amounts to is eating only as much as your system actually needs. Only you can determine that. It may take a while to learn, but it is all part of the journey.

"Every individual should, as a general rule, restrain himself to the smallest quantity which he finds from careful investigation, enlightened experience and observation will fully meet the alimentary wants of his system, knowing that whatsoever is more than this is evil." - Dr. Sylvester Graham.

3. Adhere to the proper food combination laws (see the chapter on "Guidelines that Do Not Work and Laws that Do").

4. Make sure fruits are ripe before eating them. How to tell when fruits are ready to be eaten was discussed previously.

5. Enjoy your food! If food is not enjoyed it cannot be efficiently digested. It is why I recommend using a raw vegan dipping sauce for raw vegetables, at least until the food can be enjoyed au naturel, without sauce.

6. If emotionally strung out or upset about something before eating, then skip the meal. Studies have shown that fear, anxiety, tension and anger constrict the entire digestive system and dry up the digestive juices.

7. Limit water or other fluid intake during a meal. It only dilutes the digestive juices that are needed for proper digestion. Drink any liquids at least 1/2 hour before, and typically no sooner than 1 hour after a meal. Protein and fat meals require the longest times to pass through the stomach (up to 4 hours), so adjust the consumption of liquids after the meal accordingly.

8. Eat to live, instead of live to eat. This was the dictum of Socrates, the most exemplary of the Greek philosophers. It represents the tried and tested way of health attained by the Greeks during the Golden Age of Athens.

"The rest of the world lives to eat, but I eat to live." - Socrates (470-399 B.C.).

Doing these things, or even only five of them, greatly assists in obtaining the health and vigor we are all seeking.

Colonics and Enemas

"Death begins in the colon." - Elie Metchnikoff.

Nutritional experts contend that many of the problems we are now facing, including age-related health disorders, are due to the condition of our colons. But they go further and tell us that many, if not most, diseases of humankind originate in the colon. This incredible assertion is explained in the books by Arnold Ehret, Dr. Ann Wigmore and Dr. N. W. Walker that are listed in the Bibliography, and is supported by other nutritional experts.

Hippocrates said, "All disease begins in the gut."

"Your constitutional encumbrances throughout the entire system are the source of every disease; the greatest and most harmful source of lowered vitality, imperfect health, lack of strength and endurance and any and all imperfect conditions. All have their source in the colon, never perfectly emptied since your birth." - Arnold Ehret, *The Mucusless Diet Healing System*.

What if we acted on this information? If there is a direct link between the diseases of humankind and the condition of the colon, shouldn't we do whatever is possible to eliminate toxic waste buildup and the plate-out of the plaque in the colon? Of course we should, and each of us can.

The Cure for Arthritis

Colonics and enemas help to remove the plaque-like deposits in our colons and release and move toxins out of our systems. In this way, they accelerate the self-cleansing and healing process of the body. Nutritional experts Arnold Ehret, Dr. Norman Walker and others consider colonics and enemas either highly advantageous or absolutely necessary for healing chronic diseases.

If you have never had a colonic or enema, you are not alone. Most people have never had them, and many have never even heard of them. However, as we journey to optimum health we become more and more our own doctors. The transition to a healthy diet, such as the raw vegan diet, is the time to learn what these procedures are and how to perform them.

Colonics (also known as colon irrigations or colon hydrotherapy), are procedures performed in the privacy of a personal suite at a local colonic establishment. They help clean out the toxins and wastes accumulated in the colon.

Colonic establishments are located in most cities. The average cost for a colonic irrigation (or hydrotherapy) ranges $60-$100 and you can purchase multiple sessions to save money. I have done the colon hydrotherapy several times. The machine is self-operated and easy to use. You can control it at your own pace for as long as you want. For me, that was about 30 minutes. I decided on the colonics after I read the books by Dr. N.W. Walker in the Bibliography, and particularly his book, *Become Younger*.

A less expensive way to help the detoxification process is to perform enemas at home. Enema kits are available at most retail stores (Wal-Mart, drug stores, etc.). Each kit has a number of small plastic bottles that contain a saline solution. The procedure is to lie down, turn on one side and insert the tip of the bottle and squeeze the bottle. I discovered that better results are obtained by replacing half of the saline solution with freshly-squeezed lemon juice, and using 2 bottles at a time instead of one.

Other types of enema kits are available, such as the travel-bag variety which consists of a long plastic tube and a plastic bag that can be hung from a door knob.

Doing enemas is a good, positive change to make in your life. It is a learning experience that many would much rather avoid, but again, you are becoming more and more your own doctor as you continue on the optimum health journey.

If you have less than three bowel movements a day then you should be doing colonics and/or enemas on a more frequent basis than once a month. Otherwise, once a month is recommended.

Colonics and enemas are not coffee-table topics for discussion. They are real-world procedures that need to be understood if anyone is serious about achieving optimum health.

For a more thorough discussion of the need for colonics and enemas, see the books by Arnold Ehret and N.W. Walker that are listed in the Bibliography.

Remember, if optimum health and longevity required no knowledge or effort or discernment whatsoever on the part of the individual, then they would be easy to come by and everyone would have them. If optimum health could be sold as a magic pill or silver bullet, anyone could easily become healthy without the slightest effort, and this book would not be written. But all things are given to us at the price of labor.

The Cure for Arthritis

"The "basement" of the human "temple" is the reservoir from which every symptom of disease and weakness is supplied in all its manifestations." - Arnold Ehret, *The Mucusless Diet Healing System*.

<u>How to Fast</u>

Short-term fasts, typically of no more than 4 days' duration, may be done at home without the supervision or expense of a fasting professional. You can learn about them by reading books on fasting, such as the books on fasting that are listed in the Bibliography, including Paul C. and Patricia Bragg's book, *The Miracle of Fasting*.

It is commonly observed by those who fast regularly that after about the third day there is no longer a feeling of hunger.

Fasting is not that difficult. You get used to it very soon. It does wonders not only for the body but also for the soul. When I fast, I like to read about fasting and think about how much energy is being conserved from the high-energy demands of digestion and is being used for deep bodily cleansing and healing. Drinking pure distilled water, with or without herbal teas (such as chamomile and lavender), fills the stomach and quells hunger. I typically fast every morning, and more often when I sense the need for it. It is a wonderful learning and growing experience.

You should fast when you can detect your body's signals to fast. It is then that you should fast. However, if you have a serious health condition, then you should jump into fasting right away.

The first fast is a real learning experience, and there will be hunger pangs because of eating habits. But Nature knows best. Fight the 4-6 meals a day habit and try fasting whenever you are ready for it. You won't die, and it will be a new experience for you, a richly rewarding experience that only you will know about.

"It is requisite that men should live up to the simplicity of nature, which teaches us to be content with little, and accustom ourselves to eat no more than is absolutely necessary to support life, remembering that all excess causes disease and leads to death." - Luigi Cornaro, *How to Live 100 Years, or Discourses on the Sober Life*.

You should have a goal or objective for the fast, such as to remedy a health issue or fight a disease. If you think about the goal when fasting, it will help you to complete the fast.

I try to fast often to give my digestive organs a break. The longest duration fast for me was 5 days, during which time I ingested only distilled water or herbal teas in distilled water. I broke the fast because I didn't see any need for prolonging it since I had already been on the raw vegan diet for some time and enjoyed good health by the continued self-cleansing that an exclusive diet of raw plant foods provides. However, whenever my body tells me to abstain from foods, I will fast.

I recommend that fasting be practiced regularly like all other aspects of the raw vegan diet. In my opinion, all raw vegans should perform at least a 2-day fast periodically, drinking only distilled water or herbal teas in distilled water during those two days. When the time is right, which is typically when the body has been on the self-cleansing diet for a year or more, we should learn how to fast. Fasting produces a profound and beneficial effect on the nerves as well as the psyche and health of the individual.

A type of fasting that may be practiced at every meal is eating less during meals, such as ending meals when we are two-thirds full. It's a skill that you can learn which promotes genuine health.

The Cure for Arthritis

"Your fasting is always pleasing in the eyes of the angels of God. So give heed to how much you have eaten when your body is sated, and always eat less by a third." - Attributed to Jesus, *The Essene Gospel of Peace, Book One*.

One of the things fasting does is make us more cognizant of what we are putting into the body. It makes us more aware of the quality and quantity of the foods we eat. It also makes us more aware of what food combinations are doing us harm.

I recommend the books on fasting by Herbert M. Shelton, Paul C. and Patricia Bragg, Arnold Ehret, Paavo Airola and Professor Spira (see Bibliography). They cover most aspects of fasting and describe everything one needs to know about how best to perform fasts, especially the first fast. These books clearly reveal that fasting should be a way of life in order to escape the many of the ways of death.

The big myth is that we have to eat a lot to be healthy.

Each of the above-recommended books on fasting has recommendations on how long one should fast. Take Paul C. Bragg's book for example. He recommends progressing as follows (my remarks are added):

1. At first, do a weekly fast of 24-36 hours. *You learn a great deal on the very first fast. Fasting gets easier as you continue.*

2. After maintaining the weekly fast, do a 3-4 day fast in addition to the weekly fast. *These fasts are very effective in dissolving deep-rooted, accumulated toxins.*

3. After fasting as recommended above for about 6 months, add in a 7 day fast.

4. After about a year of continuing the above fasting program, do a 10 day fast.

Arnold Ehret in his book, *The Mucusless Diet Healing System*, states that the most exact and unerring diagnosis of a person's overall health condition is how they respond to a short fast. The more quickly a person feels worse during a short fast, the greater are his encumbrances and the worse is his overall health condition.

Ehret recommends starting at first with the no-breakfast plan, then following up with a 24-hour fast, learning as you go. Then gradually increase up to 3, 4 or 5-day fasts, while between fasting providing and rebuilding the body with the best raw materials, such as found in mucusless foods (raw fresh fruit, leafy greens and non-starchy vegetables). Such an intermittent fasting program will gradually improve and regenerate the blood and dissolve and eliminate deposited wastes from the deepest tissues of the body.

"All the vitality and all the energy I have comes to me because my body is purified by fasting." - Mahatma Gandhi.

Fasting assists the body's self-cleansing process which helps us attain optimum health. When the body is sufficiently cleansed of the poisonous waste materials that have accumulated in it from years of wrong eating, then comes true health, health as you may have never experienced it before. We need to use fasting, as well as colonics and enemas, to purify our bodies of the filth that has accumulated in them from years of wrong eating.

Each fast is a new adventure, a break from the almost constant digestion that occurs in the body, a time when all the organs of the body take a very needed break, and, just as importantly, a break from the daily routines and behavior patterns we all strive to maintain.

Before your first fast, I recommend changing your diet to a whole plant food diet, such as the raw vegan diet. You can jump into the diet directly, or transition to it from whatever diet you may be on as explained in many of the books in the Bibliography, such as *The Powers That Heal*.

Fasting causes a marked improvement in an ill-health condition. But the efficacy of fasting in curing ailments depends on the individual's eating habits and how long they have been practiced. It also depends on the duration of the fast. According to fasting care professionals, relief from excruciating pain, such as from rheumatoid arthritis, can be had within only a few days of beginning a fast, but longer fasts are often required to completely eradicate the disease.

"However, this kind does not go out except by prayer and fasting."
- Jesus in the Bible, Matt. 17:21.

The healing process can be speeded up depending on what is done to assist it. For example, if you periodically fast and perform colonics and/or enemas, then quicker results can be expected. If you do not do these things, then delayed results can be expected. But the important thing is, the healing process begins in earnest when you are committed to the whole plant food diet.

Persistence, willpower and patience are often required for natural cures to be effective. Fasting is one of the ways they can be learned.

My Story

I first noticed a pain in my left hand while driving the car. I thought I had sprained it somehow. At that point, about nine years ago, I was not convinced that I had arthritis. However, after about a month of the pain, I suspected that it was more than just a sprained wrist. Then I went online to search for the answers.

Based on what I read on the Internet, I realized that I had arthritis. The pains increased monthly, although they would subside for short periods of time. Soon, it was constant pain, even while in bed, and I couldn't do anything about it except just take it, or so I thought at the time.

Supplements

The websites I polled for what should be done for arthritis recommended taking various supplements. Many supplements are offered for arthritis. Some of the websites recommended taking calcium supplements, because the body needs calcium to build strong bones and to avoid osteoporosis.

My diary became the journal of my progress in battling arthritis. Based on my journal notes, it was not long after the pains of arthritis developed in my hand that I took 500 mg tablets of calcium twice a day, and 500 mg of magnesium oxide and zinc supplements twice a day. Only later did I find out that these supplements can worsen an arthritic condition because inorganic minerals, the kind found in almost all mineral supplements sold today, are not properly utilized by the body, but can get deposited in the joints and tissues of the body, as described in this book.

The Cure for Arthritis

After being on the calcium supplements for about a month, I noticed that the arthritis had spread to both hands, and there were times when the pains spiked in intensity, or flared up. The arthritis also spread to my feet, including the toes, and, unknown to me at the time, the lower spine. But not knowing any better, I continued taking the calcium supplements for several months, believing that they were doing me good.

I visited doctors and chiropractors who X-rayed the joints and confirmed arthritis in the above-indicated locations.

After months passed, I stopped taking the calcium supplements and began taking glucosamine sulfate (GLS), and boron supplements, which, according to their producers, and also some websites, are supposed to relieve the pains and inflammation of arthritis.

Web articles claim that GLS can regenerate cartilage, and that boron can relieve the pains of arthritis and assist the body in utilizing calcium, phosphorus and magnesium. Trusting in the claims of these sources, I took 500 mg of boron and 500 mg of GLS supplements twice daily, and continued to do so until I realized that they were not improving my condition.

While GLS is a non-mineral supplement, boron, like calcium found in supplements, is an inorganic mineral. Boron supplements are typically made from boron glycinate, and glycinate (magnesium glycinate) is also an inorganic mineral.

I also tried avocado soybean unsaponifiable (ASU) in tablet form, and methylsulfonylmethane (MSM) and cetyl myristoleate (CMO), in capsule form.

The Cure for Arthritis

The supplements are known to be somewhat effective in relieving the symptoms of arthritis for a certain percentage of people, as shown in controlled clinical trials conducted by the laboratories that manufacture the supplements. However, the supplements are also known to be completely ineffective based on clinical trials conducted by independent laboratories. Nevertheless, I gave each of them sufficient time to work on my condition. The result was the same, I experienced no improvement.

It is noted that, according to the Web, ASU is a natural product derived from vegetables, MSM is a crystalline compound that contains 34% organic sulfur that is found in fruits and vegetables, and CMO is a fatty acid found naturally in certain animals, including mice, cows, beavers, and whales. Since CMO contains animal products, it probably contributes to bodily acidity and/or toxicity, two causes of arthritis as explained in this book.

The overall result of taking the supplements described was that I was no closer to a permanent cure for my condition than the day I started searching for a cure, except that I gained experiential knowledge about what remedies did not work for me.

In addition, I know now that many of the claims made for supplements on the market are not rational in light of what nutritionists tell us about the body's inability to assimilate inorganic minerals. By taking these supplements, I believe that I was unwittingly adding fuel to the fire, because I believe that I was already getting enough of these minerals, such as calcium and boron, from the whole plant foods I was consuming at the time.

Again, I strongly suspect that some of the supplements did more damage to my joints and the rest of my body than existed before I started taking them. Also, as supported by the notes I took at the time, they were, even with wishful thinking thrown in, of no help for my condition.

Then, the bones of the affected joints began to increase in size (bone deformities). I now believe that the bone deformities that developed may well have been prevented, or at least lessened in severity were it not for the inorganic mineral supplements I took in the first year of my arthritis. However, I have learned that I'm not the only one who has made matters worse for themselves by trusting Web articles about what should and should not be done for arthritis.

I talked to doctors, as well as other arthritics, about what might be done to heal my condition, but instead of taking the palliative measures that they recommended, including pain killers, I was looking for a cure.

I tried everything I knew to lessen the pains, giving each remedy sufficient time to work on my condition. Some of the remedies seemed to work to a certain extent, but none of them relieved the pains or the inflammation of my condition. It seemed that I went through practically every so-called "cure" for arthritis in my search, as is documented in this book.

All of this took time, but the result was that I came away realizing that no one really knew the answers, and that all I got for my efforts were recommendations or theories about how to treat my condition, but no sure cure. I was close to giving up the search and concluding that the doctors were right, that a cure for arthritis did not exist, because as far as I could tell no one really knew how to cure it.

I knew that I wasn't born with arthritis, but that it developed over a period of years before the pains became noticeable, and all the while it was doing its destructive work in my body. I also knew, from the books I read and the people I talked to, that if I did nothing about my condition, it would only get worse. It was obvious that a new approach was required if I was to cure my arthritis. Maybe it had something to do with abiding by Nature's laws, as some of the books indicated.

I did not give up the search. I discovered other books about arthritis that talked not about the various ways of curing arthritis through supplementation, but curing it by other means.

My experiences with alternative medicine treatments for arthritis are now discussed.

Refined Salt

I had used table salt on my foods for most of my life. Then when I became aware of its dangers to the heart, I switched to "sea salt." But, like table salt, it was a refined product that had been heated to high temperatures and bleached white in color. Its chemical structure was altered, and it was not the right kind of salt to consume, as shown in this book. I kept getting painful cracks at the corners of my lips.

According to a 2009 Warren King website,[32] cracking at the corners of lips is explained as due to an excessive consumption of salt, baked foods or saturated fats. Since I wasn't eating a lot of baked foods or saturated fats at the time because I had adopted the vegetarian diet, it was apparently due to the salt. When I cut down on my salt intake, the cracks went away.

---

[32] Article entitled, "The Intestines-Diagnosis: Our Mouth Speaks Eloquently of the Small Intestine."

The Cure for Arthritis

As explained previously in this book, many nutritionists and nutrition-minded medical doctors believe that ingesting refined salt, such as table salt, is harmful to the body. It can also worsen the symptoms of arthritis.

As mentioned previously in the chapter on "How to Change the Situation," Dr. Ann Wigmore stated emphatically in her book, *Be Your Own Doctor*, that she cured herself of arthritis by eliminating table salt from her diet.

At first, I avoided foods that have a high salt content, such as pizza sauce, and canned soups and vegetables. I also avoided high-salt condiments, such as mustard and ketchup. As a result, the flare-ups of the pains became less in a matter of days, both in their intensity and duration. However, if I returned to these food products, the flare-ups would return. This went on for a while, but eventually it made me change many of the ways I was eating.

Seeing encouraging signs, I excluded all table salt and refined sea salt from my diet for a period of four months to see what effect it would have on my condition. The ban included not purchasing or eating any canned, jarred or bottled food products that listed "Salt" or "Sea Salt" in the ingredients, and not using table salt or refined sea salt on any of my foods. During this time, the only salts I received were those contained naturally in plant foods. I saw improvement in my condition, especially in the left hand and right big toe.

As I continued to read about salt, I began using natural sea salt, such as Celtic Sea Salt or Real Salt, which I still use and believe is beneficial to health. It is typically available in whole food stores and on the Web. I found that natural salts had no adverse effects on my condition. I used these salts mostly in colloidal form, as explained in the chapter on "Salt."

The Cure for Arthritis

<u>Niacin (Vitamin B3)</u>

I tested niacin on myself for several months using 25-250 mg of niacin. I took the following forms of niacin daily, one form at a time, for about two months: Only the first form causes the flush.

Niacin, 25 mg.

Niacinamide, 250 mg.

Inositol Hexaniacinate, 200 mg.

I can testify how uncomfortable the niacin flush is. It is like having a medium to bad sunburn on the face, neck and head, but deeper than the skin, lasting about 40 minutes. Not only does it feel like a sunburn, it looks like it. Fortunately, like other B vitamins, niacin is not stored in the body but is soon flushed out through the eliminative organs.

I gave each form of niacin what I considered to be sufficient time to work on my condition. However, none of them relieved the pains or the inflammation. But that is no reason why others should not try niacin therapy to see if it works for them.

The niacin caused me more disappointment because no perceptible improvement in the pains or inflammation of my condition was discernable from it. It may have been because I was not using a large enough dosage, which, in addition to being on a healthy diet, is required for the niacin cure to be effective, as noted in the chapter on "The Importance of Alternative Medicine."

The Cure for Arthritis

Nightshades

In the search for the cure for arthritis, I read an article on the Web that linked arthritis to nightshade vegetables. The article led me to Dr. Norman Childers' book, *Arthritis -- Childers' Diet That Stops It!*, which advocates eliminating all nightshades from the diet. Included in the book are testimonies of individuals who were completely cured of their arthritis by avoiding nightshade foods.

As discussed previously, nightshades are plants that contain solanine and/or nicotine, chemicals that for hundreds of years have been known to cause arthritis in grazing animals.

Nightshades include tobacco, tomatoes, potatoes (white, yellow and red potatoes, but not sweet potatoes), eggplant, peppers (except for black and white pepper), paprika and lesser known foods.

Having lived in the American Southwest, I was accustomed to eating Mexican-American foods, which include tomatoes and hot chili peppers. Also, I have loved eating potatoes all my life. A typical meal for me would include potatoes and hot-salsa. Therefore, this new information was difficult for me to put into practice. But after I read the book, I gave it a try.

For a period of about nine months, I eliminated all nightshade vegetables from my diet. Since I had already stopped smoking, nicotine was not a concern. For potatoes, I switched from white, yellow and red varieties to sweet potatoes, because they are not of the same plant family as the other potatoes. However, I experienced little or no improvement in my condition. But again, just because a certain therapy did not work for me does not mean that it will not work for others.

The Cure for Arthritis

It was difficult, from a purely scientific standpoint, to do all the things I did to lose my pains and inflammation in isolation from each other. It was simply not possible to isolate all the different the things I did to see what each alone would have done for my condition due to my zeal to cure my condition. So, many of the things I did were done together with other things. However, taking that into account, after eliminating all nightshades from my diet there was no perceptible improvement in my condition.

The fact that the no-nightshades diet did not work for me was a great disappointment because, from reading Childers' book, I had expected my pains and inflammation to disappear slowly, but surely, within the 9 months, and especially since it indicated that for my condition, which according to the book was a rather advanced case that included bone deformities, it would typically require 9-12 months of no-nightshades to see relief.

After the trial with the no-nightshades diet, I hungered once more for chili peppers and tomatoes, and when I tried some organic varieties for over a week, there were absolutely no adverse effects on my arthritis.

Not everyone has the same sensitivity for foods, but from the experience, I must conclude that I do not have sensitivity for nightshades that many people do have.

It leads me to believe that many of the cures that are attributed to the no-nightshades diet may be achieved simply by cutting back on foods that cause *acidity* in the body, which, as discussed in this book, include fast foods and restaurant foods, that almost always include nightshade vegetables in the forms of French fries, baked or mashed potatoes, and ketchup, together with the many high-protein meat and dairy products that are served in these establishments.

Nevertheless, that is only an opinion. It may well be that after reading Dr. Childers' book, the reader may feel it is their duty to eliminate nightshades from their diet to find out whether they are sensitive to these foods. It is entirely possible, based on the testimonies in the book, that this treatment alone will eliminate many people's symptoms.

Herbs and Spices

Many books about arthritis promote or accentuate the taking of certain herbs and spices to cope with the pains and inflammation of arthritis. The books have reported that such plant substances, taken in powdered, tablet or capsule form, have varying degrees of success in lessening the pains and inflammation of arthritis. However, based on my research, many of these claims have been made by none other than the pharmaceutical companies that manufacture these supplements.

Nevertheless, to see what effect herbs and spices would have on my symptoms, I took for months, ginger and turmeric, two spices that are said to reduce arthritis symptoms. I took them separately, and in combination with each other. Ginger proved to be of little or no help in lessening my pains, so I discontinued it. Turmeric gave me gastric trouble, so I discontinued it too.

I then tried Boswellia in capsule form, which I took before or after meals. However, Boswellia also gave me gastric trouble.

I also tried other herbs, such as burdock, stinging nettle, cat's claw and devil's claw. Some of these supplements came in capsules and others in tablet. These substances caused me to experience either a headache or an upset stomach, so I discontinued them.

The Cure for Arthritis

Another spice I took was cayenne pepper (a nightshade vegetable) in powdered form, which I used on my foods at most meals. While cayenne pepper did not lessen my symptoms, it did boost my overall health in various ways, so I still use it on my foods. I believe that this spice has many health benefits, many of which are reported on the Web. One of the benefits is that it can cure hemorrhoids, as documented in the book on hemorrhoids listed in the Bibliography.

The negative results I received from taking the aforementioned herbs and spices could have been because I wasn't using them in large enough quantities, or I had stopped their use before any relief of the pains and inflammation could be seen. However, it is my opinion that if positive feedback is not received by the body on any food that is eaten, no matter what the type or variety -- fruit, vegetable, Superfood, herb or any other kind of food -- then that food should either be eaten in a more ripe condition, in smaller quantities, in proper combinations with other foods, or it should be avoided. The body is no fool. It recognizes foods that disagree with it or do it harm by giving warning signals. Our job then is to correctly interpret these signals.

Cider Vinegar

I discovered a book that made more sense the more I got into it. It was *Arthritis & Folk Medicine* by Dr. D. C. Jarvis. The book described how apple cider vinegar (ACV) can cure arthritis.

Dr. J. C. Jarvis, a Vermont physician who practiced in the days following WWII, cured many of his arthritic patients by prescribing diluted apple cider vinegar with honey, taken twice daily at or between meals. He claimed that arthritis was caused by the buildup of calcium deposits, and possibly other mineral deposits, in the joints and tissues of the body, and that ACV effectively dissolve these deposits back into the bloodstream for their elimination.

When I learned how osteoarthritis is closely linked to inorganic calcium deposition in the joints, I began taking ACV and honey in the recommended proportions, which are 1-2 tablespoons of ACV and 1-2 tablespoons of honey in a glass of water.

I used raw, unpasteurized and unfiltered ACV, either Bragg's or a similar product, sold in whole food stores. As explained previously, it contains the "mother," which is a murky substance found at the bottom of the bottle that contains enzymes and nutrients. Just shake up the bottle to get the enzymes and nutrients dispersed in the ACV. For honey, I used raw, organic and unfiltered honey sold in whole food stores, to get the full health benefits of the honey.

I read on the Web that some people take ACV straight, without adding water or honey. I decided to see if it would speed up the dissolving process by releasing more of the trapped calcium and other minerals into the bloodstream for their elimination.

I steadily increased the concentration of ACV until it was 1/3 ACV to 2/3 water, which I took with honey for about a month. It was a strong drink. It resulted in irritating the esophagus to where I had a continual hoarse throat, which was not due to a cold, flu or other infections but was solely due to the high concentration of the ACV. I observed no improvement in my condition from the higher concentrations.

I re-read Dr. Jarvis's books and reduced the concentration back to the recommended amount. The hoarse throat soon went away.

The Cure for Arthritis

The lesson learned was that using higher than recommended concentrations of ACV causes excess acidity in the body, which is one of the things we are trying to prevent with the cure. Again, if ACV is mixed with water in a higher proportion than that recommended, it will cause an acidic condition.

When I began taking the ACV drink, I used regular water from the municipal water supply (i.e., faucet water). But when I read Dr. Norman W. Walker's book, *Water Can Undermine Your Health*, and Paul and Patricia Bragg's book, *Water, The Shocking Truth That Can Change Your Life*, which warned of the harmful health effects of drinking regular (mineralized) water, I changed to distilled water.

As discussed in the chapter on "The Importance of Alternative Medicine," regular water contains inorganic minerals, such as calcium. This is especially true if you live in areas of the country that have large deposits of limestone, like where I lived. Since one of the causes of arthritis is calcification (mineralization) of the joints, we should minimize our intake of inorganic minerals of all kinds, including calcium. Even many bottled waters, the source of which is typically a municipal water supply, contain over a gram of minerals like calcium. For a more complete discussion of the health benefits of drinking distilled water, see the chapter on "Distilled Water."

When I switched from faucet water to distilled water in the ACV drink, it took only about 3 weeks to see my arthritis flare-ups diminish. With continued use, together with the other parts of the cure, the pains continued to subside until they were no longer noticed. The bone enlargements (deformities) still existed, but the pains went away. It gave me new hope that a complete cure for my condition, including the bone deformities, would be possible.

The Cure for Arthritis

When the pains subside, you may want to stop taking the ACV drink. From my experience, you will know when to stop from signals the body gives as explained in the previous section, including the diminishing of the pains.

If the pains return after ceasing the ACV drink, it probably means that your diet has not improved to where it should be in reducing the intake of foods and substances that cause toxic acid and mineral deposits to form in the joints and tissues of the body. It indicates that you should continue with all parts of the cure until the process is completed.

We are all good learners, and we adapt to what we learn very readily. You can heal yourself of arthritis, but you must first clean out the abundance of toxic wastes that have accumulated in your system over a lifetime of harmful eating practices.

Persistence and patience took me there, and they will take you there too. In about 6 months, the pains in my hands and toes had subsided to where I almost never noticed them.

<u>Healthy Diets</u>

I know now from what I learned about arthritis that I was mainly responsible for the pains and inflammation of my condition because I helped bring them about by ingesting the foods and substances of an ordinary diet for many years.

But before I reached that conclusion, I started looking more closely at my diet. Based on the books I read that talked about what really causes arthritis, I learned that the body begins to show signs of disease (not only of arthritis, but all kinds of disease) when it becomes overloaded with substances that are found in foods that the body considers to be poisonous or toxic. The books, which are listed in the Bibliography, explained that many of the substances we ingest get deposited in the joints and tissues of the body, as explained in this book. But, at the time, it was new information to me, and it took a while for it to sink in.

I will mention three books that were influential in getting me to eat healthier foods. The first was by Ann Wigmore, *Be Your Own Doctor,* which gave me new hope and became the turning point for the dietary change that would heal me of arthritis. The book reveals how importantly foods affect health, for better or worse, and how they can enable the body to heal itself of practically any health disorder. From then on, I read every book I could that discussed the direct relationship between foods and nutrition and health.

Secondly, there was Paavo Airola's *There is a Cure for Arthritis.* The book describes various natural treatments for arthritis that have been practiced for many years in the renowned health clinics of Europe and this country. The cures require not a single practice, but a combination of practices, such as healthy dieting and fasting.

The third book that helped me to shift eating habits to healthier foods was Harvey Diamond's book, *Living Without Pain.* The book is easy to read and tells how the symptoms of many widespread diseases and health issues, such as arthritis, fibromyalgia, lupus and chronic fatigue syndrome, may be significantly relieved through the self-healing process when certain foods and substances are avoided, and healthier foods are eaten.

One of the major obstacles in the way to successfully attaining a whole plant food diet is what I call the curse of "food convenience." Our society is built on fast foods and fast drinks. We need to break away from these things. It requires shifting our focus to healthy foods and drinks, those with health-appeal rather than taste-appeal. It means taking the time required to shop at local food stores for our foods, even though doing so typically takes only minutes more than it does to drive through a fast food place. This may be a major shift in thinking for many people. It's hard to break old habits. However, they were formed by repetition and they can be broken by repeatedly refraining from them.

It was only after adopting the raw vegan diet that my health really improved. After being on the diet for only a short time, not only my arthritis, but many of the other ill-health conditions I had disappeared, and I found myself for the first time in years with a surplus of energy. Just as significantly, my health continues to improve on the diet.

An aspect of a whole plant food diet that strikes me as being most interesting is that it doesn't leave you guessing about whether your health is going to improve. Your health does not stall or level-off and then decline on the diet, as it does on other diets. It continues to improve. Each day on the diet is an ongoing progression, a new adventure, sometimes trying until the key points discussed in this book are mastered, but never a losing proposition. Each day that you are on the diet you are a winner.

Raw plant foods give us the zest and energy we always wanted to have but never could quite obtain. They make us feel good about each and every day of our lives. A whole plant food diet, like the raw vegan diet, literally transforms you into a new person. Other diets cannot do this.

As discussed in the chapter on "The Importance of Alternative Medicine," results of many dietary studies, some of which are backed by the latest scientific understanding about foods and nutrition, and the wealth of knowledge that is now available that indisputably links improper diet with diseases and other health issues, all point to the importance of eating a whole plant food diet, such as the raw vegan diet, for promoting and sustaining health.

An important concept to include in one's thinking about foods is that they are a source of medicine as well as nourishment. When this concept is internalized, great strides are possible in health.

"Let food be thy medicine and medicine be thy food." - Hippocrates.

Some people will not eat fruit because the last time they did, it caused them too much discomfort. Most likely, it was because the fruit was eaten in an un-ripened condition, or else it was combined improperly with other foods. For example, when dates or figs are eaten with pineapple, the result may be a stomachache, because sweet fruit (dates and figs) should not be eaten with acid fruit (pineapple)." See the chapter on "Guidelines that Do Not Work and Laws that Do."

Fasting

I consider fasting to be instrumental to the attainment of true health, even if it means just skipping a meal occasionally or practicing the no-breakfast plan.

The history of fasting and its many benefits to human health were discussed in the chapter on "The Importance of Alternative Medicine." As explained therein, fasting acts so powerfully on the body that many diseases can be completely cured through its practice alone. For this reason, I highly recommend that some type of fasting, even if it is just eating less during meals, be regularly practiced if the aim is to achieve and maintain optimum health.

It is worthy to repeat what was stated previously in a footnote. If fasting can cure almost all human diseases, then what does that tell us about how diseases and other health disorders originate? Doesn't it clearly indicate that the principle cause of health disorders lies in the foods that are eaten? Does it not assuredly implicate improper diet as the main cause of many of our ailments?

Fasting is so significant to the attainment of genuine health that if the reader gets nothing out of this book but the importance of fasting, then the book will have served its purpose, because, as previously mentioned, fasting signifies, and in the practice of fasting is found, almost all of the health principles that are elucidated in this book.

Exercising the Joints

It was well after I first noticed the pains and inflammation of arthritis that I began exercising the affected joints. I elected to do so after reading about how exercising the joints may help break up the hard acid and mineral deposits in the joints.

I pulled and twisted my arthritic joints twice daily, doing exercises I learned from the Web, and shook my hands and fingers vigorously twice a day. It was, at first, painful and slow going. But as with the practices of the cure kicked in, it became less painful.

I haven't stopped exercising my joints. I believe that it is a proactive or preventive measure, like drinking distilled water, to ward off joint stiffness and other degenerative effects as we age.

The Cure for Arthritis

More About the Cure

The prognosis is excellent for anyone who takes the cure, not only for improvements in the symptoms, but for general health and well-being.

Since I began taking the cure over three years ago, the pains and inflammation of arthritis I suffered for over seven years have not returned, and there have been no new joints in my body that have fallen to the disease. My life, to a great extent, has returned to normal, and I'm enjoying many things that I thought would never be possible for me again.

Once the basics of the whole plant food diet are understood (and they are understood when they are put into practice), you have at your disposal the most potent healing and transformational tool ever available. And that is when the adventure really begins.

On a whole plant food diet, self-cleansing is in full gear. The self-cleansing process begins internally and is then reflected externally. This goes against conventional wisdom which says that to be clean all you must do is thoroughly wash with soap and water, but that only contributes to external cleansing. Internal cleansing is necessary to remove the toxins and pasty crud that have accumulated in the organs and tissues of the body from years of eating cooked and starchy foods and other foods and food products that are harmful to health. Normal signs of detoxification, previously discussed, are likely to be experienced, especially as more raw fruits and vegetables are eaten.

The skin, and particularly the skin of the face, reflects our internal health condition. A bad skin complexion (for example, pimples or blotches on the face) indicates internal poisoning. A clear complexion reveals internal health. It doesn't take long on a whole plant food diet like the raw vegan diet for the skin of the face to clear up, and then become smoother.

Some people spend large amounts of money on beauty products and preparations. If the money were spent instead on self-education about foods and nutrition, and on raw, organic fruits, vegetables, leafy greens and other living plant foods, it would allow health and youthful appearance to be attained without the aid of these products.

As stated previously, want to look young? Eat raw plant foods. Want to look old? Eat cooked foods.

Health improvements reported by raw food eaters the world over have included not only the complete healing of diseases, but changes indicative of rejuvenation, such as wrinkles disappearing, improved vision, hair growing back and hair color returning to that of former years, among other things. These signs, while seemingly miraculous, are logical consequences of eating living plant foods once you understand the healing powers of these foods. Such improvements are due to the life force in raw plant foods, life force made available to anyone on the raw vegan diet.

On the raw vegan diet, the body is cleansed not only of poisonous substances that have accumulated over the years and have been deposited deeply in body tissues, but also those that get into the body from the environment, or from foods and drinks, such as chlorine and heavy metals from municipal drinking water, pesticides in non-organic produce, and tobacco and alcohol use.

"Any substance, when taken into the body, is either a food or a poison." - Dr. Herbert M. Shelton, *Superior Nutrition*.

The Cure for Arthritis

Modern nutritional experts believe that fruits and leafy green vegetables are the greatest cleansers of the body. Both food groups cause toxins to be released from the tissues. The more fruits and leafy greens we eat on a regular basis, the more our internals are scrubbed clean and the more our outward improvements are manifested. Since the self-cleansing process will be on-going from now on, so will visible health improvements.

The effectiveness of the self-cleansing process is also evident by the composition, odor and frequency of stools. Bowel movements become smoother, less smelly and more frequent, which are all signs of internal cleansing becoming a more normal process, and indicating a less clogged up condition due to better digestion and the ongoing removal of poisons from the body. On the raw vegan diet, you may find that the number of bowel movements per day is at least as many as the number of meals eaten per day. Constipation is unknown on the raw vegan diet.

To avoid arthritis from taking root in the body again, remember the statement made by Paavo O. Airola, N.D., (quoted previously):

"A person recovering or recovered from arthritis should always be careful with acid-forming foods: bread, cereals, animal proteins, cheese, etc. It is imperative to continue with the program of vital nutrition long after recovery if lasting results are to be expected." - Paavo O. Airola, N.D., *There is a Cure for Arthritis*.

The Cure and Longevity

The cure for arthritis cleanses the body of its toxins and impurities so dramatically that it literally sets the stage for the possibility of a longer life.

Alchemists, scientists and laymen throughout history have tried to discover the secrets of longevity. It was once believed that all one had to do was to find the "Elixir of Life," which was thought to be a certain food or mixture of foods that would bestow eternal youth on its possessor.

The Holy Scriptures appear to be the origin of the belief that there once was an Elixir of Life. In Genesis 1:29, God gave to mankind a diet consisting of whole plant foods, which is best described as the raw vegan diet. But there were two trees in the Garden of Eden that had special fruit; one was the tree of good and evil, and the other was the tree of life, a tree that would make man live forever.

Genesis 2:9:
"And out of the ground the Lord God made every tree grow that is pleasant to the sight and good for food. The tree of life was also in the midst of the garden, and the tree of the knowledge of good and evil."

Genesis 3:22:
"Then the Lord God said, "Behold, the man has become like one of Us, to know good and evil. And now, lest he put out his hand and take also of the tree of life, and eat, and live forever --.''

The Cure for Arthritis

Genesis 3:24:
"So He drove out the man; and He placed cherubim at the east of the garden of Eden, and a flaming sword which turned every way, to guard the way to the tree of life."

Many seekers of long life have wondered what kind of food grew on the Tree of Life. As far as we know, no one has succeeded in identifying it or, what is probably the same thing, the Elixir of Life. But sometimes beliefs are hard to dispel, especially when they are based on truth.

Everyone wants to live longer, whether for putting things to right or for enjoyment. However, not everyone knows how to go about ensuring their longevity.

One of the great contributors to our understanding of how to live a long life was Luigi Cornaro, a nobleman who lived in Italy during the fifteenth and sixteenth centuries. His remarkable books include *Sure Methods of Attaining a long and Healthful Life*, *The Surest Method of Correcting an Infirm Constitution,* and *How to Live 100 Years, or Discourses on the Sober Life*. The books are listed in the Bibliography.

The term that Cornaro used in his books to describe how to attain long life through optimum health was "sobriety". By sobriety he meant the following:

"Sobriety is reduced to two things, quality and quantity. The first consists in avoiding food or drinks which are found to disagree with the stomach. The second, to avoid taking more than the stomach can easily digest." - Luigi Cornaro, *How to Live 100 Years, or Discourses on the Sober Life.*

The Cure for Arthritis

According to his books, Cornaro ate very sparingly each and every day of his life, after curing himself in his 40s of maladies that his doctors said would soon cause his death. In his later years he never overate, but always under-ate.

As discussed in the chapter on "How to Change the Situation," immediately after the Flood, when animal food was permitted to be eaten, the average human lifespan fell from about 900 years to about 400 years. Today, according to the latest worldwide statistics, the average human lifespan is 72 years. What does this indicate? It indicates a slow decline in human longevity based on a departure from the God-given diet of Genesis 1:29.

"And God said, "See, I have given you every herb that yields seed which is on the face of all the earth, and every tree whose fruit yields seed; to you it shall be for food." - Gen. 1:29.

Luigi Cornaro lived to 102. What does it tell us about the importance of reducing the quantity of food that we eat, as well as fasting between meals which he obviously did by eating so sparingly? According to his books, Cornaro never needed spectacles (glasses), his hearing remained unimpaired, and he could climb hills effortlessly until he died. And he kept his mind sharp by learning new things.

In the last two hundred years, many investigators have studied extended human lifespans by visiting various cultures of the world. They have tried to ascertain why certain peoples lived longer than others. They have performed clinical studies and determined that the centenarians (those who were at least 100 years old) had the following things in common.

- They were moderate or light eaters
- They ate very little butter or salt

- They ate little, if any, meat
- They ate fresh foods
- They kept up strenuous activity throughout their lives
- They liked to do outside work and rose early

"The major characteristic of the diet of longevous people is low total calorie intake throughout life." - Dan Georgakas, *The Methuselah Factors*.

Some of the clinical studies we have of extended human lifespan are documented in the books that are listed in the Bibliography, including *The Methuselah Factors* by Dan Georgakas, *Youth in Old Age* by Alexander Leaf, and *Healthy Aging* by Andrew Weil.

It was only during the last century that nutritionists concluded that the closer an organism (animal or human) comes to its minimal daily food requirements, the longer its lifespan will be. But God was ahead of everyone. He prescribed the quantity of daily food intake in Exodus Chapter 16. Each person was to eat no more than an omer of manna per day. An omer is an ancient unit of volume measurement equal to about 2 quarts. According to the Bible, it is best for us to eat no more than 2 quarts of food per day.

Dr. N.W. Walker, whose books are listed in the Bibliography, spent most of his life exploring man's capability to extend life. He lived to be 99 according to the Web, but some sources say 109. His books are referred to several times in this book since they provide much insight into what foods should be eaten for longevity and optimum health.

According to Dr. Walker, the foods that people should eat for longevity are the foods of the raw vegan diet. Raw plant foods are the most conducive of any foods to longevity because they contain an abundance of life force properties and enzymes and do not contain man-made or -altered ingredients.

Maybe we are only now beginning to understand how to achieve longevity. As discussed in the chapter on "Dangers to Avoid," enzymes are important life catalysts that are abundant in raw plant foods. Dr. Ann Wigmore, whose books are listed in the Bibliography, believed that enzyme preservation is the secret to longevity.

"Enzymes, apparently, are the key to longevity; they seem to neutralize the basic causes of aging and enable the body to retain its youthful qualities." - Dr. Ann Wigmore, *Be Your Own Doctor*.

It is our duty to strive for optimum health while we remain in the world of the living. No one knows the day of their death. Happily, we have nothing to do with that date; only God knows its appointed time. But we must be good stewards of our lives and do what is right to promote and sustain our health.

If you seek to extend the term of your existence, then adopt the raw vegan diet, keep physically and mentally active and do not overeat.

Afterwards

The cure imposes limits on gratifying our desires for certain foods, and disproves the cultural imposed belief that supplementation is necessary for heath, but it does not restrict our lives. Rather, it frees us from becoming the slaves of harmful food habits and cravings and the irrational use of supplements.

When the pains and inflammation of arthritis have gone away, there may be a tendency to return to one's former ways of eating, even though the dangers of doing so are well known. But even returning to supplements, such as those that contain inorganic minerals as a filler material or the main ingredient (such as calcium supplements), will likely cause the return of the pains and inflammation that the diet has thwarted. Fortunately, the body gives us many feedback signals that can be used to keep us on the right track.

However, to retain the great benefits that have been gained, we must keep our distance from commonly consumed foods, drinks and substances that cause arthritis. An essential part of wisdom is knowing what we cannot adequately handle. By learning about foods and nutrition and becoming more and more familiar with the practices that are described in this book, we gain the wisdom to keep ourselves in health.

My advice is simply to keep with a whole plant food diet, such as the raw vegan diet, watch the substances that you ingest that contribute to the causes of arthritis, and, if you flounder here and there and the symptoms of arthritis reappear, just return to the diet and the other practices.

Next Steps

Those who change their diets as described in this book profit in numerous ways other than curing themselves of arthritis. They know an abundance of health that was never known before.

The information presented in this book may be extended beyond the scope of arthritis to other diseases and health issues, including other diseases that end with "itis," such as bursitis and colitis.

I encourage you to read the books listed in the Bibliography. They have much to offer the novice as well as the long-time student of foods and nutrition. We all like to eat, but it is only when we learn to eat foods that promote health, not destroy it, that our health flourishes. The books provide valuable information and inspiration that will help all seekers of health. They have been a constant source of encouragement to me on my health journey. Take the time to delve into them and you will be glad that you did.

It should be remembered that, as Paavo O. Airola, N.D., says in his book *There is a Cure for Arthritis*," the most distressing fact about arthritis is that millions of sufferers are given no hope for a cure or any relief from their discomfort and misery. When cured of your arthritis, consider helping others cure themselves of the disease. Give them the hope they need and deserve.

In Closing

The best preparation for tough times ahead is how we deal with the difficulties encountered today. This book has described how to deal with some of the most perplexing and challenging issues that can ever confront any of us. Were we to acknowledge that everything bad that happens to us is an opportunity in disguise, a lesson to be learned for our benefit and a way of strengthening us in some way, then our trials and tribulations would be much easier to bear and we would be better able to see the intended purpose for them.

We're not likely to get the answers we need to improve our health from conventional medicine practitioners. Conventional medical training allows for little, if any, instruction on how the body heals itself when it is deprived of foods and drinks that do it harm and provided with the foods and drinks it needs for health. In addition, it takes a while for conventional medicine to recognize the benefits of treatments that do not employ their approved methods, and even longer to put such treatments into practice. Therefore, each of us must make the difference in our health by solving as many health problems as we can. We find the answers we are looking for when we dig hard enough for them.

The feelings of exuberance and goodness that result from the eating raw plant foods, and combining them properly, are the opposite feelings experienced on ordinary diets because of poor nutrition, poor digestion and constipation. The life force properties of raw plant foods make all the difference.

As more and more fad diets, miracle treatments and supplements become available and attract the attention of millions, so are more and more people throughout the world discovering the health advantages of eating at variance with the customs of the times, and the simple truth that eating natural plant foods leads to good health. They are taking back responsibility for their health and abandoning culturally accepted foods. Truly, these are the lucky ones.

In taking the cure for arthritis and, particularly, in adopting the whole plant food diet, sufferers of arthritis are preparing for themselves a great springtime of health that will affect their lives in extraordinary ways for many years to come.

Bibliography

The following books were the major resources used to write this book.

1.. Dr. Norman F. Childers, Arthritis - Childers' Diet That Stops It! 2006.

2. Paavo O. Airola, N.D., There is a Cure for Arthritis, 1968.

3. Harvey Diamond, Fit for Life Not Fat for Life, 2003.

4. Harvey Diamond, Living Without Pain, 2007.

5. Dr. D. C. Jarvis, Folk Medicine, 1958.

6. Dr. D. C. Jarvis, Arthritis & Folk Medicine, 1960.

7. Margaret Hills, Treating Arthritis: The Drug-Free Way.

8. Robert O. Young and Shelly R. Young, The pH Miracle, 2010.

9. Paul C. and Patricia Bragg, Apple Cider Vinegar, Miracle Health System, 2008.

10. Paul C. and Patricia Bragg, The Miracle of Fasting, 2005

11. Dr. Edward Howell, Enzyme Nutrition, 1985.

13. Paul C. and Patricia Bragg, Water, The Shocking Truth That Can Save Your Life, 2004.

14. Abram Hoffer, Andrew W. Saul and Harold D. Foster Niacin, The Real Story, 2012.

15. T. Colin Campbell, The China Study, 2006.

16. Dr. Michael Greger, How Not To Die, 2015.

17. John Smith, Fruits and Farinacea- The Proper Food of Man, 2015.

18. Russell T. Trall, Scientific Basis of Vegetarianism, 1970.

19. Dr. Caldwell Esselstyn, Jr., Prevent and Reverse Heart Disease, 2007.

20. Jethro Kloss, Back to Eden, 2014.

21. Dr. Ann Wigmore, Be Your Own Doctor, 1982.

22. Dr. Ann Wigmore, Why You Do Not Have to Grow Old, 1985.

23. Dr. Ann Wigmore, The Sprouting Book, 1986.

24. Arnold Ehret, The Mucusless Diet Healing System, 2015.

25. Arnold Ehret, Physical Fitness Through a Superior Diet, Fasting, and Dietetics , 2018.

26. Arnold Ehret, Rational Fasting and Roads to Health and Happiness, 2002.

27. Arnold Ehret, The Cause and Cure of Human Illness, 2001.

28. Teresa Mitchell, My Road to Health, 1987.

29. Norman W. Walker, Colon Health, 2005.

30. Norman W. Walker, Become Younger, 1978.

31. Norman W. Walker, Fresh Vegetable and Fruit Juices, 1978.

32. Norman W. Walker, Diet and Salad Suggestions, 1985.

33. Norman W. Walker, Water Can Undermine Your Health, 1995.

34. Norman W. Walker, The Natural Way to Vibrant Health, 1972.

35. Norman W. Walker, The Vegetarian Guide to Diet and Salad, 1985.

36. Victoria Boutenko, Green for Life, 2005.

37. Victoria Boutenko, 12 Steps to Raw Foods, 2005.

38. David Wolfe, The Sunfood Diet Success System, 2008.

39. David Wolfe, Longevity Now: A Comprehensive Approach, 2013.

40. David Wolfe, Superfoods, the Food and Medicine of the Future, 2009.

41. Professor Spira, Spira Speaks, Dialogs and Essays on The Mucusless Diet Healing System, 2014.

42. Dr. Bernard Jensen, Guide to Diet and Detoxification, 2000.

43. Dr. Bernard Jensen, The Healing Power of Chlorophyll, 1973.

44. Fred S. Hirsch, Internal Cleanliness, 1987.

45. Tonya Zavasta, Beautiful on Raw Uncooked Creations, 2005.

46. Kristina Carrillo-Bucaram, The Fully Raw Diet, 2016.

47. Karyn Calabrese, Soak Your Nuts, 2011.

48. Herbert M. Shelton, Superior Nutrition, 1994.

49. Herbert M. Shelton, Fasting Can Save Your Life, 1978.

50. Herbert M. Shelton, Food Combining Made Easy, 1982.

51. Dr. Russel Blaylock, Excitotoxins, The Taste that Kills, 1997.

52. Joe Alexander, Blatant Raw Foodist Propaganda, 2005.

53. Horst Kornberger, Global Hive: Bee Crisis and Compassionate Ecology, 2012.

54. Annie Payson Call, Power Through Repose, 1905.

55. Steve Meyerowitz, Sprouts, The Miracle Food, 1997.

56. Dr. Henry Lindlahr, Philosophy of Natural Therapeutics, 1975.

57. Dan Georgakas, The Methuselah Factors, 1980.

58. Alexander Leaf, M.D., Youth in Old Age, 1975.

59. Andrew Weil, M.D., Healthy Aging, 2005.

60. Luigi Cornaro, Sure Methods of Attaining a long and Healthful Life, 1660.

61. Luigi Cornaro, The Surest Method of Correcting an Infirm Constitution, 1660.

62. Luigi Cornaro, How to Live 100 Years, or Discourses on the Sober Life, 1660.

63. Dr. Johnny Lovewisdom, Dietetics Vitarianism, 2001.

64. Gabriel Cousens, M.D., Conscious Eating, 2000.

65. Jeffery M. Smith, Genetic Roulette, 2007.

66. F. Batmanghelidj, M.D, Your Body's Many Cries for Water, 2008.

67. Dr. Allen E. Banik, The Choice is Clear, 1989.

68. Robert Morse, N.D., The Detox Miracle Sourcebook, 2004.

69. Arnold Paul De Vries, Therapeutic Fasting, 1958

70. Dr. Kristine Nolfi, M.D., The Miracle of Living Foods, 1981.

71. T. Colin Campbell and Howard Jacobson, Whole: Rethinking the Science of Nutrition, 2014.

72. Wallace D. Wattles, Health Through New Thought and Fasting, 2007.

73. Francoise Wilhelmi de Toledo, MD, and Hubert Hohler, Therapeutic Fasting: The Buchinger Amplius Method, 2018.

74. Edward Hooker Dewey, M.D., The No-Breakfast Plan and the Fasting Cure. 1900.

75. Edward Hooker Dewey, M.D., The True Science of Living. 1894.

76. Upton Sinclair, The Fasting Cure, 1911.

77. Hereward Carrington, Vitality, Fasting and Nutrition, 1908.

79. Herbert M. Shelton, Health for the Millions, 1968.

80. O. L. M. Abramowski, Fruitarian Diet and Physical Rejuvenation, 1916.

81. Prof. Arnold Ehret's Mucusless Diet Healing System: Annotated, Revised, and Edited by Prof. Spira, 2015.

82. Sergei and Valya Boutenko, Eating Without Heating, 2002.

83. The Natural Hygiene Handbook, 1996.

84. NIH (National Institutes of Health) Record, April 2015.

85. G. Edmond Griffin, World Without Cancer, 2004.

86. Rich Anderson, Cleanse & Purify Thyself, 2000.

87. Howard F. Lyman, Mad Cowboy, 1998.

88. Eckhart Tolle, The Power of Now, 1999.

89. Stan Shepherd, Raw Veganism, 2018.

90. Stan Shepherd, The Powers That Heal, 2019.

91. Stan Shepherd, Stop Sciatica and Spinal Stenosis, 2019.

92. Stan Shepherd, How to Completely Get Rid of Hemorrhoids Naturally: A Permanent Cure, 2019.

93. Stan Shepherd, A Christian Diet, 2019.

About the Author

S. H. Shepherd, 71, has researched and studied the human health field for over 30 years. An engineer by training, he has witnessed the rapid decline of health in this country over the years due to commonly eaten foods. He has also witnessed the erosion of joint mobility and quality of life of many people who have been stricken with arthritis. He cured his arthritis by the cure that is presented in this book.

Appendices

Appendix I, Berg's Tables

Appendix II, The Dirty Dozen and The Clean Fifteen

Appendix I, Berg's Tables

Berg's Tables[33] list what foods are acid-binding and acid-forming. The terms are synonymous with mucus-binding and mucus-forming, respectively.

The larger the "plus" or "acid-binding" value, the more the mucus-binder or eliminator the food is. The larger the "minus" or "acid-forming" value, the more the mucus-producer the food is.

According to these tables, meat and grain products are the most acid-forming foods, whereas fruits and vegetables are the most acid-binding foods. In other words, meat and grain products are the most mucus-producing foods, whereas fruits and vegetables are the most mucus-eliminating foods.

---

[33] Data taken from the tables published in Arnold Ehret's book, Mucusless Diet Healing System, and the tables available on the Web at the time of this writing.

The Cure for Arthritis

Name of Food	Plus or Acid-Binding	Minus or Acid-Forming
Flesh		
Meat (Beef)		-38.61
Chicken		-24.32
Ham, Smoked		-6.95
Meat (Beef)		-38.61
Mutton		-20.30
Bacon		-9.90
Ox Tongue		-10.60
Pork		-12.47
Rabbit		-22.36
Veal		-22.95
Fish		
Herring, Salted		-17.35
Oysters	+10.25	
Salmon		-8.32
Shellfish		-19.52
Whitefish		-2.75
Eggs		
Eggs, Whole		-11.61
Eggs, White		-8.27
Eggs, Yolk		-51.83
Milk & Milk Products		
Butter, Cow		-4.33
Buttermilk	+1.31	
Cream	+2.66	
Lard		-4.33
Margarine		-7.31
Milk, Cow	+1.69	
Milk, Goat	+0.65	
Milk, Human	+2.25	
Milk, Sheep	+3.27	
Milk, Skim	+4.89	
Swiss Cheese		-17.49

Name of Food	Plus or Acid-Binding	Minus or Acid-Forming

Grains and Grain Products

Barley		-10.58
Black Bread		-8.54
Cakes (White Flour)		-12.31
Cornmeal		-5.37
Farina		-10.00
Graham Bread		-6.13
Macaroni		-5.11
Oat Flakes		-20.71
Oat Flour		-8.08
Oats		-10.58
Pumpernickel Bread	+4.28	
Quaker Oats		-17.65
Rice, Polished		-17.96
Rice, Unpolished		-3.18
Rye		-11.31
Rye Flour		-0.72
Wheat, Refined		-8.32
Wheat, Whole		-2.66
White Bread		-10.99
Zwieback		-10.41

Vegetables

Asparagus	+1.10
Artichoke	+4.31
Cabbages	+4.02
Cauliflower	+3.09
Chicory	+2.33
Dandelion	+17.52
Dill	+18.36
Endives	+14.51
Green Beans	+5.15
Kohlrabi Root	+5.99
Milk, Skim	+4.89
Leeks	+11.00
Lettuce, Head	+14.12
Mushrooms	+1.80

Name of Food	Plus or Acid-Binding	Minus or Acid-Forming
Red Cabbage	+2.20	
Red Onions	+1.09	
Rhubarb	+8.93	
Spinach	+28.01	
String Beans (Fresh)	+8.71	
Watercress	+4.98	

Root Vegetables

Black Radish, with Skin	+39.40	
Celery Roots	+11.31	
Horseradish	+3.06	
Red Beets	+11.33	
Sugar Beets	+9.37	
Sweet Potatoes	+10.31	
White Potatoes	+5.90	
White Turnips	+10.80	
Young Radish	+6.05	

Fruits

Apples	+1.38	
Apricots	+4.79	
Banana	+4.38	
Blackberries	+7.14	
Cherries	+2.57	
Cucumbers	+13.50	
Currants	+4.43	
Dates, Dried	+5.50	
Figs	+27.81	
Grapes	+7.15	
Lemons	+9.90	
Olives	+30.56	
Oranges	+9.61	
Peaches	+5.40	
Pears	+3.26	
Pineapple	+3.59	
Plums	+5.80	
Pomegranates	+4.15	

The Cure for Arthritis

Name of Food	Plus or Acid-Binding	Minus or Acid-Forming
Prunes	+5.80	
Pumpkins	+0.28	
Raisins	+15.10	
Raspberries	+5.19	
Sour Cherries	+4.33	
Strawberries	+1.76	
Sweet Cherries	+2.66	
Tangerines	+11.77	
Tomatoes	+13.67	
Watermelon	+1.83	

Nuts

Acorns	+13.60	
Almonds		-2.19
Chestnuts		-9.62
Coconut	+4.09	
Hazelnuts		-2.08
Walnuts		-9.22

Legumes

Beans, dried		-9.70
Lentils		-17.80
Peanuts		-16.39
Peas		-3.41
Soy Beans	+26.58	

Drinks, Sweets

Cocoa		-4.79
Chocolate		-8.10
Tea leaves	+53.50	
Coffee	+5.60	

Appendix II, The Dirty Dozen and The Clean Fifteen

Several years ago, the Environmental Working Group (EWG) published lists of fruits and vegetables known as the Dirty Dozen and the Clean Fifteen. These lists indicate foods with the most and least pesticide residues on them based on data compiled by the USDA. The lists are updated annually. They reflect pesticide residues found on foods after they were washed with water.

The Dirty Dozen

The foods highest on this list have the most pesticides on them.

1. Strawberries
2. Apples
3. Nectarines
4. Peaches
5. Celery
6. Grapes
7. Cherries
8. Spinach
9. Tomatoes
10. Sweet bell peppers
11. Cherry tomatoes
12. Cucumbers

According to EWG, buying organic for the twelve fruits and vegetables on this list can reduce our pesticide exposure by at least 90 percent!

The Clean Fifteen

The foods highest on this list have the least pesticides on them.

1. Avocados
2. Sweet corn
3. Pineapples
4. Cabbage
5. Sweet peas (frozen)
6. Onions
7. Asparagus
8. Mangoes
9. Papayas
10 Kiwi
11. Eggplant
12. Honeydew melon
13. Grapefruit
14. Cantaloupe
15. Cauliflower

There is no need to buy organic for the fruits and vegetables on this list, except for cabbage (number 4) and papayas (number 9). For cabbage, according to David Wolfe's book, *The Sunfood Diet Success System,* non-organic cabbage has large amounts of pesticides are used on it. Papayas are GMO foods and have pesticides on them.

Some types of produce are more prone to containing pesticides residues than others. Avocados, sweet corn and pineapples, for example, are not so prone because of their protective outer layer of skin. Not the same for strawberries and other berries.

Index

A

Acidity, 39-40, 45, 68-74, 88, 106, 118, 120, 126, 130, 137, 141, 148, 169-170, 172, 192, 199, 202.

AGEs (advanced glycation end-products), 98, 134.

Anemia, 173-174.

Arthroplasty, 25-26.

Arthrodesis, see Joint Fusion.

Arthroscopy, 23-24.

ASU, avocado soybean unsaponifiable, 194.

B

Boswellia, 200.

Blood pressure, 37, 47, 56, 107, 118, 149, 173.

Bursitis, 11, 17, 45, 69, 83.

C

CAFOs, Confined Animal Feeding Operations, 67.

Calcium, 14, 43-47, 68. 74-82, 83, 121, 124, 151, 153, 156, 192-194, 203-205, 218.

Calcification (mineralization) of the joints, 49, 74-82, 88, 122, 205.

Cartilage, articular, 13-17, 19-20, 23, 25, 69, 74, 80-82, 84, 86, 129-131, 194.

Chlorophyll, 84, 103, 106. 172.

CMO, cetyl myristoleate, 194.

Colitis, 11, 56, 69.

Colonics, 140, 183-186, 191-192.

Cooked foods, dangers of, 40-42, 69, 71, 73-74, 93, 97-98, 104, 109-110, 118-119, 132-139, 141-142, 146, 161, 172, 212.

Constipation, 29, 39-40, 85-86, 88, 99, 112, 132-133, 139-141, 148, 213, 221.

D

Detoxification, 29, 72, 108-112, 117, 128, 186, 211.

Diets

    American (traditional), 40, 70, 91, 113, 117, 144, 159, 161.

    No-nightshades, 53, 201.

    Vegetarian, 96-99, 102.

    Vegan, 96-99, 102.

    Raw vegan, 96-99, 107, 109, 111-113, 117, 139, 157-158, 166-167, 182, 184-187, 190, 207, 210-213, 216-218.

    Whole plant food, 37-49, 68-74, 87, 92, 95, 104, 107-111, 113, 116-120, 121-123, 126, 130-131, 151, 172, 176-178, 184, 193, 197, 207, 211, 213, 218, 221.

Digestion, general, 42, 46, 54-55, 59, 69, 106, 136, 165-169, 184-187, 191, 194, 215, 223. Also, see Enzymes.

Distilled water, 44, 49-51, 77, 97, 154-159, 189-190, 207, 212.

Drugs, 19, 29-31, 47, 54, 57, 68, 84-85, 111, 119, 128, 183, 189.

E

Enemas, 183-186, 191-192.

Enzymes, 34, 40-42, 45-46, 48, 68, 71, 98, 104, 106, 112, 119, 132, 134-139, 142, 146-147, 185, 204, 218.

Excitotoxins, 36-37, 85.

F

Fatigue, 47, 55, 86-87, 110, 136, 181, 207.

Fasting, 53-63, 96-97, 140, 147, 192, 207, 211-212, 29.

Food combinations, 71, 127, 146, 163-168, 176, 181, 189.

Food Pyramid, 159-163.

Fusion, see Joint Fusion.

FDA, 20, 22, 101.

Fibromyalgia, 16, 207.

G

Ginger, 200.

Gluttony, 142.

GLS, glucosamine sulfate, 194.

GMO foods and food products, 67, 85, 100-102, 238.

Gout, 9, 11,16, 45, 63, 81, 88-90.

H

Hard acid deposits, 34, 47, 69, 71, 73, 90, 124-125, 212.

Health information controlled, 59, 70, 160

Herbs and spices, 202-203.

Hemorrhoids, 203.

Honey, 43, 47-49, 119, 124, 126, 138, 205-206, 207.

Hyaluronic acid (hyaluronan), 21-22.

I

Immune system, 19, 21, 85, 106, 113, 116-117.

Indigestion, 71, 127, 146, 163-168, 176, 181, 189.

Inorganic minerals, see Minerals, inorganic,

"Itis" diseases, 17, 84, 219.

J

Joints, 11-26, 81, 130, 156, 193-214.

Joint arthroplasty / joint replacement, 25-26.

Joint Fusion, 17-18, 23, 25-26.

Juvenile arthritis, 16.

K

Knee Replacements, 19, 23-26.

L

Lupus, 16, 207.

M

MSG (Monosodium Glutamate), 36, 71, 85.

MSM, methylsulfonylmethane, 194-195.

Minerals, inorganic, 35, 38, 49-51, 76-82, 88, 97, 122-124, 152, 154-157, 195, 197, 205-206, 221.

N

Nightshade vegetables, 52-53, 200-201.

No-nightshades diet, see Diets.

NSAIDs, 12, 18-22.

Nutrients, 31, 34-35, 39, 41-41, 45, 48, 67-68, 70-71, 74, 78, 87-88, 98-99, 104, 109, 113-114, 116, 121, 132, 134, 137, 140, 143-144, 174-176, 206.

Nutritional deficiency, 66-68, 74, 87-88, 174.

O

Obesity, 15, 135, 142-144, 164.

Oils, fractionated, 131.

ORAC rating of foods, 114-116.

The Cure for Arthritis

Osteoarthritis, 19-20, 22-26, and elsewhere throughout this book.

Osteoporosis, 74-76, 78, 121, 193.

P

Pesticides, 84, 100-102, 154, 212, 235-236.

Plate-out, of deposits,185.

Psoriatic arthritis, 9, 16.

R

Radiation, 27, 29, 113.

Raw vegan diet, see Diets.

RDAs (Recommended Daily Allowances), 73-75.

Rheumatoid arthritis, 9, 16, 25, 30, 45, 48, 73, 190.

S

Saturated fats, 36, 104, 128-130, 140, 197.

Self-cleansing (see Detoxification).

Starchy foods, 82, 84, 98,107, 131, 137-140, 145, 159, 165, 168-169, 190, 212.

Steroids, 12, 18, 21.

Superfoods, 69, 104, 112, 114, 169, 203.

Supplements, 32, 34, 66, 73-79, 83, 86-87, 107, 113, 115, 120-121, 193-196, 202, 210, 219-220, 222.

Surgery, 12, 18, 22-27, 29, 32, 56-57.

T

Tobacco, 51, 199, 212.

Toxicity, 19, 23, 38, 83-87, 98, 106, 110, 119, 125, 130, 137, 141, 195.

Turmeric, 202.

U

Uric acid, crystals, 62, 80-81, 86-88.

USDA, 20, 68, 75, 101, 114, 160, 162-163, 235.

V

Vegan diet, see Diets.

Vegetarian diet, see Diets.

W

Whole plant food diet, see Diets.

Willpower, 91, 177, 180, 192.

Made in the USA
Columbia, SC
09 December 2020